Epilepsy Explained

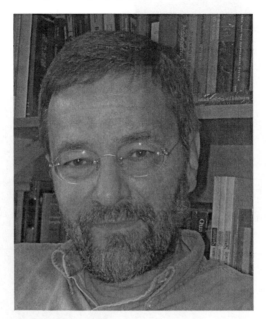

In memory of Ulrich Altrup (1944–2007)

EPILEPSY EXPLAINED

A Book for People Who Want to Know More

Markus Reuber, MD, PhD, MRCP
Senior Lecturer in Neurology
University of Sheffield
United Kingdom

Steven C. Schachter, MD
Professor of Neurology
Harvard Medical School and
Director of Research, Department of Neurology
Beth Israel Deaconess Medical Center
Boston, MA

Christian E. Elger, MD, PhD, FRCP
Professor of Epileptology
University of Bonn
Germany

Ulrich Altrup, MD
Professor of Experimental Epileptology
University of Münster
Germany

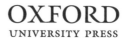

OXFORD
UNIVERSITY PRESS

2009

OXFORD
UNIVERSITY PRESS

Oxford University Press, Inc., publishes works that further
Oxford University's objective of excellence
in research, scholarship, and education.

Oxford   New York
Auckland   Cape Town   Dar es Salaam   Hong Kong   Karachi
Kuala Lumpur   Madrid   Melbourne   Mexico City   Nairobi
New Delhi   Shanghai   Taipei   Toronto

With offices in
Argentina   Austria   Brazil   Chile   Czech Republic   France   Greece
Guatemala   Hungary   Italy   Japan   Poland   Portugal   Singapore
South Korea   Switzerland   Thailand   Turkey   Ukraine   Vietnam

Published by Oxford University Press, Inc.
198 Madison Avenue, New York, New York 10016

www.oup.com

Library of Congress Cataloging-in-Publication Data

Epilepsy explained: a book for people who want to know more /
Markus Reuber ... [et al.].
    p.   cm.
1. Epilepsy—Popular works.   I. Reuber, Markus.
RC372.E6645 2009
616.8′53–dc22
2008030606
ISBN-978-0-19-537953-2

The science of medicine is a rapidly changing field. As new research and clinical experience
broaden our knowledge, changes in treatment and drug therapy occur. The authors and
publisher of this work have checked with sources believed to be reliable in their efforts to
provide information that is accurate and complete, and in accordance with the standards
accepted at the time of publication. However, in light of the possibility of human error or
changes in the practice of medicine, neither the author, nor the publisher, nor any other party
who has been involved in the preparation or publication of this work warrants that the
information contained herein is in every respect accurate or complete. Readers are encouraged
to confirm the information contained herein with other reliable sources, and are strongly
advised to check the product information sheet provided by the pharmaceutical company for
each drug they plan to administer.

Printed in the United States of America
on acid-free paper

To our patients

PREFACE

Epilepsy is one of the most common disorders of the brain. In addition to the effects of seizures and medications, anxiety and prejudice toward people with epilepsy can make life harder than it needs to be for those with the condition. In this book, we provide information about all aspects of epilepsy. We wrote this book for people with epilepsy, as well as for their families, friends, teachers, and caregivers, and the general public.

Our book has been written so that it does not need to be read from cover to cover. It can be opened on any page and will still make sense. We recognize that this means that some facts are repeated in different sections but felt that it was important that readers should be able to directly turn to those parts of the book most relevant to them.

This book has grown gradually over the last 10 years. It would never have been completed without the tireless enthusiasm of Ulrich Altrup, who started the book after he had designed a series of posters about epilepsy, which were shown at a German epilepsy center. Sadly, Dr. Altrup did not live long enough to see the final version. We hope that we have honored his vision with this first American edition.

Many other people have helped us with this book. We are especially grateful to Dr. A. Hecker, Dr. M. Finzel, Dr. J. von Oertzen, Dr. S. Ried, Dr. U. Specht, Professor E.-J. Speckmann, and Professor P. Wolf. We also thank L. Vollmert and G. Jakobs (supported by Professor M. Herrenberger) from the Department of Design at the Polytechnical University of Münster, Germany, who produced the drawings of people with epilepsy and their seizures.

Sheffield, Boston, and Bonn

August 2008

Markus Reuber,

Steven C. Schachter, and

Christian Elger

vii

CONTENTS IN BRIEF

CONTENTS IN DETAIL

Epilepsy Explained

1

Epilepsy: A Problem with the Brain

1.1 EPILEPSY IS A COMMON CONDITION

ANYONE CAN DEVELOP EPILEPSY

Anyone can develop epilepsy, and about one in a hundred people does. This makes epilepsy as common as diabetes or rheumatoid arthritis. However, people talk much less about epilepsy than about these other conditions.

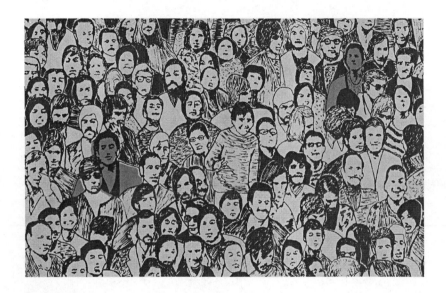

This picture shows 120 people. If they were typical of the whole population, one or two should have epilepsy. Most people with epilepsy would lead a normal life if only people without epilepsy would let them. Unfortunately, many are prejudiced about epilepsy. This book is for people with epilepsy and for people who live or work with them. It is written to inform people about epilepsy. It is meant to explain the causes and treatment of epilepsy. It is meant to be understood by everyone.

Epilepsy is as common as diabetes or rheumatoid arthritis.

EPILEPSY AFFECTS PEOPLE OF ANY AGE AND FROM ALL WALKS OF LIFE

Other medical conditions, tuberculosis for instance, particularly affect poor people. There are also diseases that are more common in rich people. Epilepsy affects rich and poor alike. A person can develop epilepsy when he or she is a baby, a young adult, or in older age.

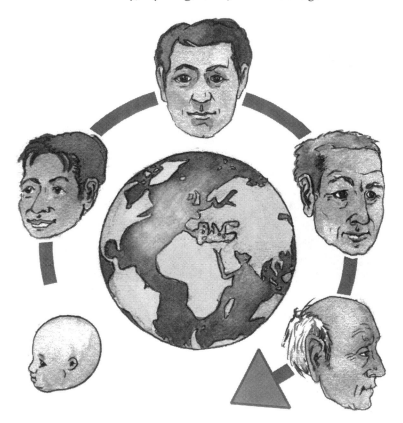

Epilepsy affects a similar number of people in all countries and cultures around the world. It has affected people for many thousands of years.

MANY FAMOUS PEOPLE HAD EPILEPSY

Epilepsy is as old as mankind. The list of famous people whom historians believe had epilepsy is overwhelming. This shows that epilepsy has nothing to do with mental disease or retardation. The list of famous people includes businessmen like Nobel, and playwrights or authors like Molière and Dostoyevsky.

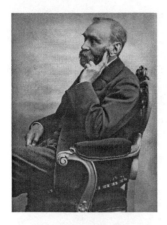

Nobel

Alfred Nobel was born in Sweden in the nineteenth century. He was a talented inventor who created a prosperous business and who made an enormous fortune from the development of explosives. These explosives were used for both peace and war. He established the best known of all prizes, the Nobel Peace Prize.

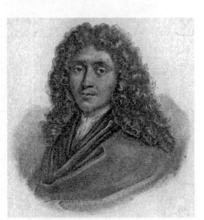

Molière

Molière is best known as a play writer. Although he lived in the seventeenth century, his comedies *Tartuffe*, *The Imaginary Invalid*, and *The Misanthrope* are still performed regularly today. He was particularly good at showing the hypocricies and follies of society through satire.

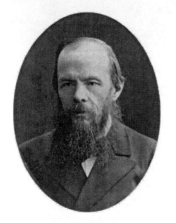

Dostoyevsky

Several of Dostoyevsky's books contain descriptions of people with epilepsy. When he wrote his books, Dostoyevsky was using his own experiences as someone suffering from epilepsy. His seizures mostly happened at night. His wife tells us how he had a seizure at a party. After this seizure, Dostoyevsky was very sad: "as if I had lost the dearest thing in my life, as if I had buried someone, this is how I felt."

EPILEPSY HAS BEEN EXPLAINED IN DIFFERENT WAYS OVER THE CENTURIES

There have been many theories about the cause of epileptic seizures. Ancient people thought they were caused by evil spirits or demons that had invaded a person's body. Others considered epilepsy a "sacred disease" thinking that people were close to God during a seizure. However, the famous Greek doctor Hippocrates knew, as long as 2,500 years ago, that epilepsy is caused by physical problems in the brain.

Hippocrates based his medical practice on observation and on the study of the human body. This made him believe that diseases have physical and rational explanations. He accurately described diseases like pneumonia and epilepsy. The knowledge and experience of Hippocrates were lost for many centuries.

Five hundred years ago, a famous book on witch hunting, the "Malleus Maleficarum," stated that seizures were a characteristic of witches. In a wave of persecution, this mistaken belief led to the death of more than 200,000 women. Many prejudices about epilepsy have survived throughout the centuries and are still present today.

For the last 200 years, epilepsy has been an area of scientific study. The first antiepileptic drug was developed about 150 years ago.

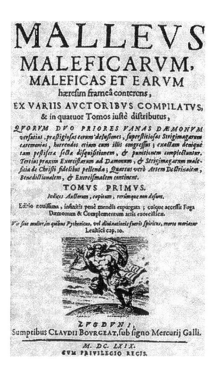

THERE ARE PEOPLE WITH EPILEPSY IN EVERY COMMUNITY

One in a hundred people has epilepsy. This means that in a town of 100,000 people, there will be 1,000 with epilepsy, and in a city of 1,000,000, there will be 10,000 with epilepsy.

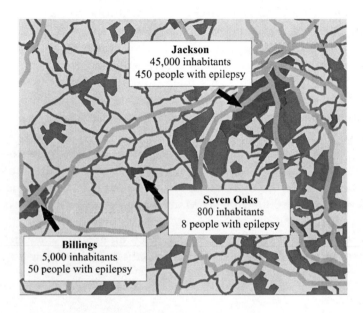

Some people join groups where they meet other people with epilepsy. Such groups (for instance the local affiliates of the Epilepsy Foundation) allow people with epilepsy to learn from each other.

The numbers under each place name show how many people in these communities have epilepsy. Doctors working in these towns and cities may know about epilepsy self-help groups. It is also possible to find out about groups using the addresses in the back of this book.

Find out if there is a support group in your area.

DOCTORS WHO TREAT PEOPLE WITH EPILEPSY

Typically, people with epilepsy have access to the support of a team of health care professionals. The person at the center of this team is the person experiencing seizures. All people on the team should communicate openly and trust each other. People with different types of expertise can join the team temporarily or permanently, such as social workers, EEG technicians, pharmacists, or surgeons. The treatment of epilepsy is usually carried out by a primary care doctor, a pediatrician, a neurologist, or an epileptologist (a neurologist who specializes in epilepsy).

Primary care doctor

More than three-fourths of U.S. adults have one physician whom they consider to be their primary physician. A primary care doctor can offer advice on a wide range of issues, from an acute illness to preventive "wellness" care.

Four years at a college or university
Four years at one of the U.S. medical schools
Doctor of medicine degree (MD)
Additional clinical training before starting independent practice

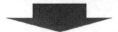

Neurologist

Neurologists are doctors with further specialist training. They are particularly qualified to treat problems with the brain and nerves. Many different conditions are treated by neurologists, and epilepsy is one of them.

Three years of further training in neurology under the supervision of a senior physician

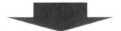

Epileptologist

Epileptologists are neurologists with special training in epilepsy.

One to three years of additional training in epilepsy.

PUBLICATIONS FOR PEOPLE WITH EPILEPSY

There is a wide range of books about epilepsy. Books provide information about epilepsy, advice on living with epilepsy, and epilepsy treatment. They are written for kids, teens, or family members and caregivers. An extensive list of books about epilepsy can be found at the back of this book.

Epileptic is a cartoonist's memoir of growing up in the 1970s in a family in which his brother's grand mal epilepsy regularly took center stage. The failure of his brother's seizures to respond to any form of treatment for any length of time or of the family to adjust to life with a chronic disease is presented in an unsentimental but straightforward way. The book is very accessible and much of it is of interest to teens.

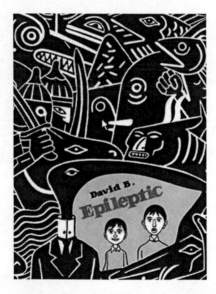

A lot of information about epilepsy is available on the Internet. "Epilepsy.com" (www.epilepsy.com) is one such website that informs people facing the diagnosis of epilepsy for the first time and people struggling with epilepsy that is proving difficult to treat.

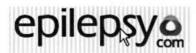
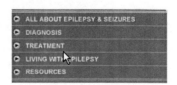

The National Institute of Neurological Disorders and Stroke provides information on epilepsy and on other neurological disorders.

ORGANIZATIONS FOR PEOPLE WITH AN INTEREST IN EPILEPSY

Many organizations across the world are dedicated to epilepsy. Most want to make the public more aware of epilepsy. They also give advice to people with epilepsy and may help them to educate their friends, family, teachers, or employers about epilepsy. All of these organizations have websites that contain information about epilepsy.

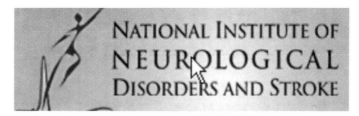

The Epilepsy Foundation is a national voluntary agency solely dedicated to the welfare of millions of people with epilepsy in the United States and their families. The organization works to ensure that people with seizures are able to participate in all life experiences. There are affiliated Epilepsy Foundation offices in nearly 100 communities.

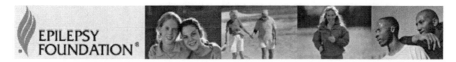

The American Epilepsy Society promotes research and education for professionals dedicated to the prevention, treatment, and cure of epilepsy. The society organizes annual conferences.

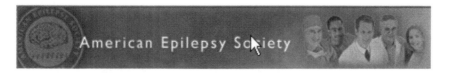

The International League Against Epilepsy (ILAE) was founded in 1909 in Budapest. It has branches in many countries around the world. It publishes the newsletter Epigraph and the journal *Epilepsia* and organizes conferences on epilepsy. Recently, the ILAE started a campaign to bring epilepsy "out of the shadows."

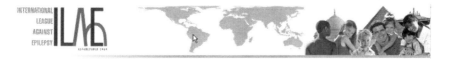

SPECIAL MEETINGS FOR PEOPLE WITH AN INTEREST IN EPILEPSY

Several epilepsy organizations have annual and sometimes worldwide meetings that bring together medical and other professionals or people with epilepsy. These meetings cover a broad range of topics, research findings, and ideas about epilepsy. Some meetings are dedicated to one particular topic, such as the long-term effects of taking antiepileptic drugs.

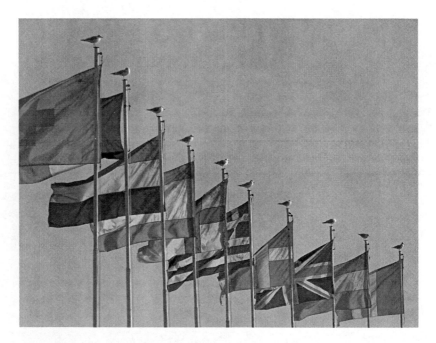

With permission from Sebastiano Gulisano

One of the most recent international epilepsy meetings focused on the following question: What induces epilepsy, and what induces seizures? The answers to these questions remain controversial. The topics that were discussed at another congress included epilepsy care, imaging of the living brain, marriage and family issues, how epilepsy develops, surgery, and the cost of epilepsy. International meetings also allow doctors to learn about new drugs for epilepsy and to discuss how to use them.

1.2 THERE ARE MANY TYPES OF SEIZURES

PEOPLE WITH EPILEPSY HAVE SEIZURES. THESE ARE SHORT INTERRUPTIONS OF NORMAL BRAIN FUNCTION

Epileptic seizures are not the only things that can briefly stop the brain from working normally or that can cause sudden movements. For example, nervous twitches of an eyelid, sudden jerks while drifting off to sleep, or trembling of the hands at times of stress are not due to epilepsy.

Sometimes it is not easy to tell whether or not a symptom, an event, or attack is caused by epileptic seizure activity in the brain. A primary care physician or specialist such as a neurologist or epileptologist should be consulted if a person may have had a seizure.

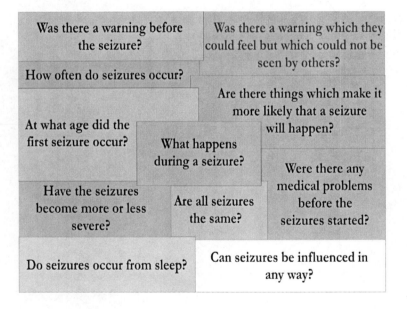

Although each seizure is slightly different, they can be divided into different types. This is the basis of a classification of seizures, which is important for choosing the best treatment.

To find out which type of seizures a person is having, doctors ask people with epilepsy many questions:

Some of these questions may need to be answered by friends or relatives who have seen a seizure. What was the first thing they noticed when the seizure occurred? Did the seizure end suddenly, or was recovery slow? Was there a period of confusion, tiredness, or unusual behavior after the seizure?

SEIZURES CAN BE CLASSIFIED IN A NUMBER OF WAYS

The classification of seizure types used at the present time has been developed over many years. Thanks to this classification, people who develop a particular type of seizure or epilepsy can benefit from the experience gained in the treatment of the same type of seizure in the past. If it is known, for instance, that a certain drug does not work for one seizure type, it makes no sense to try this drug again in someone who has just developed this same seizure type. Experience also helps to predict how epilepsy is likely to develop in someone over the years.

The classification of seizures can be likened to telling the difference between different means of transport. Although no two bicycles, cars, or motorcycles look exactly the same, it is usually not difficult to separate all bicycles from all cars or motorcycles.

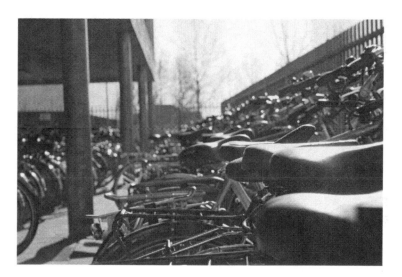

With permission from Arjen Vogel

One important classification of seizures is based on changes that can be seen in the EEG. The EEG can often tell doctors whether seizures likely come from one particular part of the brain ("partial" seizures), or whether they involve both halves of the brain from the start ("generalized" seizures).

Seizures are either "partial" or "generalized."

IN A PARTIAL SEIZURE, EPILEPTIC ACTIVITY AFFECTS JUST ONE PART OF THE BRAIN

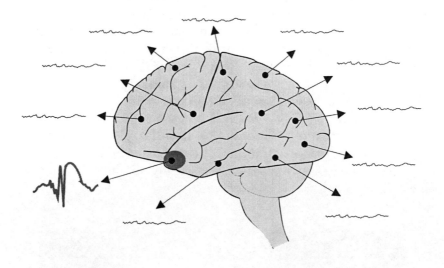

The picture shows a side view of the brain. The wavy lines marked by arrows represent the electric activity at each of the black spots, which represent EEG electrodes. The area of the brain marked in the darker shade produces abnormal electric signals that are picked up by the EEG electrodes. The EEG in this part of the brain shows spikes and waves. These are typical of the electric activity that may occur between seizures in someone with partial seizures. The place in the brain where seizures start is called the "focus." If epileptic activity during a seizure only affects the area around the focus, the seizure is called "partial" (or "focal"). The electric activity in all other parts of the brain is normal during such a seizure.

In principle, an epileptic focus can be anywhere in the brain. People with epilepsy may have one focus or more than one.

> The place where seizures come from in the brain is called a "focus."

IN A GENERALIZED SEIZURE, THERE IS EPILEPTIC ACTIVITY IN BOTH HALVES OF THE BRAIN

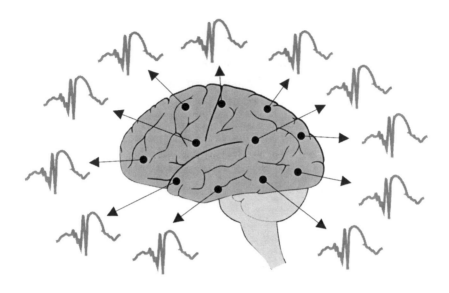

This picture shows spike-and-wave activity across the whole brain. If such epileptic activity is seen in all areas of the brain from the onset of a seizure, it is called "generalized." There are relatively subtle types of generalized seizures, such as "absence" attacks, and others that are more pronounced, such as "tonic-clonic" seizures. The fact that the whole brain is involved in generalized seizures does not mean that they are particularly difficult to treat. Often generalized seizures respond to drugs more easily than do focal, or partial, seizures.

Any partial seizure can spread from the focus after it has begun and involve the whole brain. If this happens, the seizure is called "secondary generalized." The spread of epileptic activity from a focus to the rest of the brain can take from a split second to a few minutes.

Treatment is different for partial and generalized seizures.

GENERALIZED SEIZURE: TONIC-CLONIC SEIZURE (GRAND MAL)

A tonic-clonic seizure is a major epileptic seizure. During a tonic-clonic seizure consciousness is lost and all parts of the body stiffen and jerk. A tonic-clonic seizure is frightening to see, especially the first time or if the observer is not familiar with what to do. This type of seizure has affected the way the public has thought about epilepsy for many centuries. It was often called "grand mal" in the past.

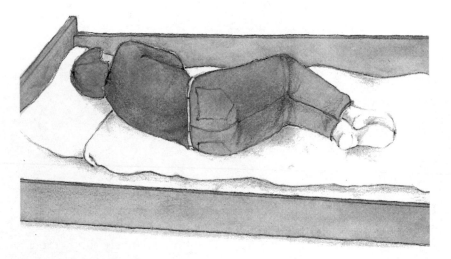

Person resting

Not everybody who has epilepsy has tonic-clonic seizures. Sometimes tonic-clonic seizures only happen during sleep. They might also happen only shortly after waking up. This would be called a "tonic-clonic seizure on awakening." Sometimes such seizures may even be provoked by lack of sleep.

At the beginning of a tonic-clonic seizure, the whole body becomes stiff. As this happens, people who are standing up fall to the ground and sometimes they scream (this does not mean that these seizures hurt; people usually cannot remember this afterwards). Next, the arms and legs begin to jerk in a regular rhythm. The jerking first becomes more violent, then it gradually subsides. During this part of the seizure, a person's complexion can look blue, they can froth from the mouth, wet themselves, and bite their mouth or tongue.

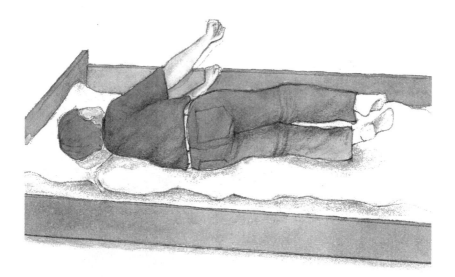

During a tonic-clonic seizure

The picture shows the first part of a tonic-clonic seizure. The body, arms, and legs are stretched out (sometimes the arms and the upper half of the body are bent). The only things some people notice about tonic-clonic seizures during sleep are saliva or blood stains on the pillow in the morning, a headache, or a sore mouth and tongue. They may also wake up having wet the bed or fallen out of bed.

GENERALIZED SEIZURE: ABSENCE SEIZURE (PETIT MAL)

"Absences" are a mild form of seizures. They used to be called "petit mal." Absence seizures consist of a short interruption of consciousness that causes people to stop briefly whatever they are doing. During this form of seizure, the whole surface of the brain produces epileptic discharges from the start to the finish. Children who develop epilepsy between the ages of 5 and 10 often have absence seizures. Research has shown that absence seizures are more common in girls, and that they can be treated easily with drugs. Once their absence seizures are treated, the children who have this form of epilepsy develop normally.

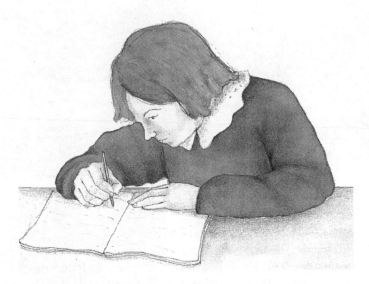

Absences may first be noticed at school. The picture shows a child trying to keep up in class.

If teachers do not know about this type of epilepsy, they often think that children are not paying attention. However, in an absence seizure, children cannot react if they are told to concentrate, and they have no memory for what goes on during the seizure.

Absence seizures are usually controllable with seizure medications. After a few years, the drugs can be stopped to see whether the seizures have disappeared. To do this, the dose of the drugs is reduced gradually. Drugs used for epilepsy should only be reduced with the help of a doctor as stopping medication can be dangerous without such guidance. Sometimes epileptic seizures flare up when drugs are stopped.

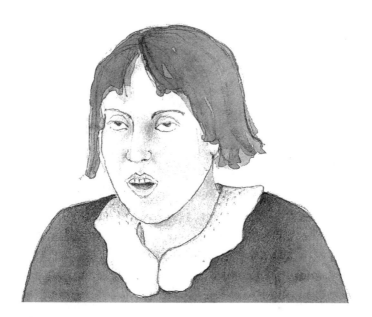

During a seizure

This girl has had a number of absence seizures in class. During these seizures, she raises her head, opens her mouth, stares straight ahead, and rolls up her eyes a little. By the time the teacher tries to get her to pay attention, the seizure is already over.

Absence seizures in children often go away after a few years.

GENERALIZED SEIZURE: MYOCLONIC SEIZURE

Myoclonic seizures are very brief jerks, typically occurring within 1 or 2 hours after waking up. Usually they last less than a second. There can be just one, but sometimes many will occur within a short time. Myoclonic seizures usually cause abnormal movements of the arms and shoulders on both sides but sometimes the whole body is affected. They usually begin in childhood, but they can occur at any age.

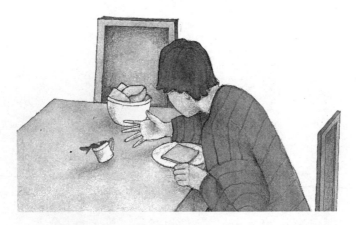

People may suddenly drop a cup or their toothbrush during a myoclonic seizure. If the legs are affected, they may fall and injure themselves. Myoclonic seizures in teens, called "juvenile myoclonic epilepsy (JME)," occur most commonly together with absence and tonic-clonic seizures.

Example

"In the morning I get these 'jumps.' My arms fly up for a second, and I often spill my coffee or drop what I'm holding. Now and then my mouth may shut for a split second. Sometimes I get a few jumps in a row. Once I've been up for a few hours, the jumps stop."

Myoclonic seizures are sometimes triggered by flashing lights or other things in the environment. Myoclonic-type movements are not always caused by epilepsy. People without epilepsy can experience such movements in hiccups or in a sudden jerk that may wake them up just as they are falling asleep. These "sleep jerks" are normal.

Myoclonic epilepsies and seizures

Juvenile myoclonic epilepsy
Progressive myoclonic epilepsy
Benign myoclonic epilepsy of infancy
Myoclonic-astatic epilepsy
Myoclonic absence epilepsy
Familial adult myoclonic epilepsy
Autosomal dominant myoclonic epilepsy
Drug-induced myoclonic seizures
Early myoclonic encephalopathy

The outlook for people with myoclonic seizures depends on the condition that has caused their seizures.

Juvenile myoclonic epilepsy, for instance, is a common form of epilepsy that is usually inherited. The seizures can be relatively easily treated with medication, but the condition does not go away on its own. Seizures must be blocked throughout life with antiepileptic drugs. In Lennox-Gastaut syndrome (LGS), which begins in early childhood, myoclonic seizures are often not blocked completely with drugs. Progressive myoclonic epilepsy is a rare form of epilepsy with a combination of myoclonic and tonic-clonic seizures. Treatment is usually not successful for very long, and people generally have more problems from their epilepsy as time goes by.

GENERALIZED SEIZURE: TONIC SEIZURE

During a tonic seizure, the muscles of the body stiffen suddenly for some seconds. Consciousness is always lost. Tonic seizures can affect the whole body or a part of the body, for instance the muscles of the shoulders and arms. Some tonic seizures are quite subtle and only cause the eyes to roll up. Most people with tonic seizures have no sensation that an attack is coming on.

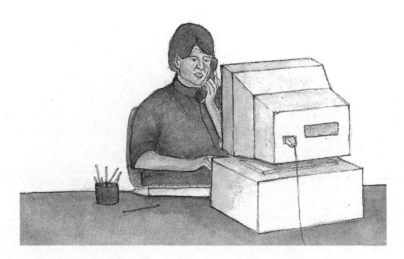

Person at work

The picture shows a woman on the telephone at work. Her tonic seizures start without warnings, so that she has no time to put down the phone. The seizures always affect the arms and shoulders, and they cause her to lose consciousness.

The woman stays in position for a few seconds and then continues to work normally. She cannot stop her muscles from stiffening up. As her legs are not affected, her seizures do not cause her to fall.

In another person, more muscles can be affected. Both arms may be raised over the head and the face shows a grimace, as if someone were pulling on the cheeks. When the muscles of the trunk are also involved, people may lose their balance and fall.

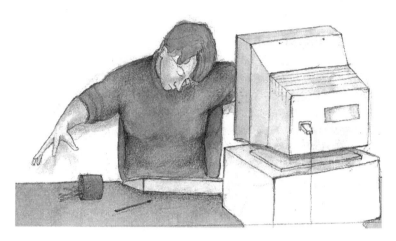

During the seizure

Tonic seizures are particularly common in a condition called Lennox-Gastaut syndrome, in which they occur with other seizure types. LGS is a severe form of childhood epilepsy. Seizures begin between 1 and 8 years of age. Tonic seizures last about 10–20 seconds. In LGS, tonic seizures most commonly occur during sleep.

GENERALIZED SEIZURE: CLONIC SEIZURE

Clonic seizures consist of rhythmic jerking movements of the arms or legs, sometimes of both and on both sides of the body. The same sort of regular twitching may also affect the face. Clonic seizures are not seen very often. They can occur at various ages, including in babies.

Brief and infrequent clonic seizures in infants usually disappear on their own within a short time. Other types of clonic seizures may need longer-term treatment.

In very young babies a harmless jitteriness can be mistaken for a clonic seizure. While seizures usually cannot be influenced, jittering stops or changes when the position of the baby's arms or legs is changed.

Toddlers sometimes have temperatures of above 105°F. When a baby's temperature is raised, clonic seizures can appear as a series of jerking movements. Each series may last only 30 seconds, but one series of jerks can follow another. In most cases, no treatment is necessary to prevent further seizures.

GENERALIZED SEIZURE: ATONIC SEIZURE

"Atonic" means without tone, and refers to the lack of tension of muscles. Another name for this type of seizure is "akinetic," which means without movement. In an atonic seizure, the head can nod when the neck muscles suddenly lose tension or people can fall to the ground if muscle tension is lost in leg muscles. Atonic seizures often begin in childhood and last into adulthood. People with atonic seizures can be injured when they fall, so they may choose to wear protection such as a helmet.

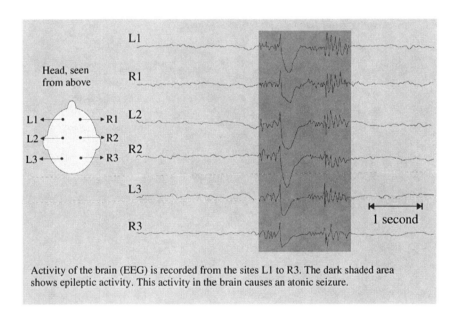

Activity of the brain (EEG) is recorded from the sites L1 to R3. The dark shaded area shows epileptic activity. This activity in the brain causes an atonic seizure.

An atonic seizure can be mistaken for a faint ("syncope"), which is a short loss of consciousness with prompt and spontaneous recovery. Syncope is caused by a brief reduction of blood supply to the brain mostly due to problems with the distribution of blood in the body. In contrast, atonic seizures are caused by a problem in the brain itself.

Seizures can only be treated successfully when their true cause has been identified.

PARTIAL SEIZURE: SIMPLE PARTIAL SEIZURE

The word "partial seizure" means that epileptic activity only affects a part of the brain. This part is also called a "focus" (this means that "partial epilepsy" is the same as "focal epilepsy"). People remain aware of what is going on during a "simple partial seizure," so they are able to recall later what happened during the seizure. In a "complex partial seizure," however, awareness is reduced and the time during the seizure will not be remembered later on.

A partial seizure starting from the dark spot causes

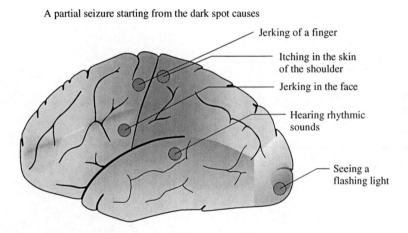

Jerking of a finger

Itching in the skin of the shoulder

Jerking in the face

Hearing rhythmic sounds

Seeing a flashing light

The symptoms or actions that happen in a simple partial seizure depend on the area of the brain in which the seizure occurs. The diagram shows a side view of the left half of the brain. Separate areas of the brain deal with vision, touch, and hearing, and movements are controlled by the area shown. Everybody's brain works like this.

In most people, it remains unclear what first causes a focus to start producing epileptic activity. However, it is important to look for possible causes of epilepsy. If the cause of seizures can be identified, it can sometimes be treated. Occasionally a seizure focus can be removed with an operation. If the focus is taken out, seizures may stop. Looking for the causes of epilepsy involves tests such as brain scans (especially magnetic resonance imaging: MRI), electrical tests (EEG, also called electroencephalography), and sometimes blood tests.

Some important causes of partial seizures

- Area of abnormal development of the brain
- Brain tumor
- Brain injury
- Infection of the brain and its lining (encephalitis or meningitis)
- Problems with the blood supply of the brain
- Parasites
- Scars

Example

Mr. C. had an accident at work. He fell off a scaffold, injured his head, and was unconscious for several days. He gradually recovered but had to spend some weeks in a hospital. Six months later, he suddenly developed partial seizures. These started with twitching of the fingers of his left hand, which spread to the whole left hand and eventually all of the left arm and shoulder. The twitching gradually stopped after 1 minute. When the twitching had stopped, the left arm was weak and heavy for a few more minutes. The accident had caused damage to the part of the brain that controls the movement of the left arm. The injury led to the development of an epileptic focus, which causes partial seizures from time to time. Mr. C. has been started on antiepileptic drugs that have reduced the number of seizures, but have not stopped them completely.

PARTIAL SEIZURE: COMPLEX PARTIAL SEIZURE

In a partial seizure, epileptic activity only affects one part of the brain, the area around the starting point or "focus" of the seizure. During a "simple partial seizure," awareness and the ability to remember things later are not reduced. During a "complex partial seizure," consciousness is reduced or completely lost. Complex partial seizures occur most commonly in those regions of the brain that are marked "frontal lobe" and "temporal lobe."

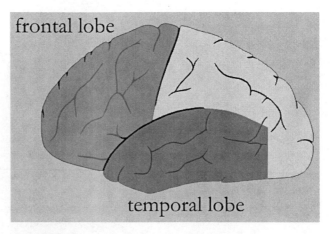

Complex partial seizures starting from the frontal lobe tend to cause movements such as jerking of the limbs, bicycling movements of the legs, pacing, or the production of hand gestures.

A complex partial seizure can cause a range of different behaviors. People may smack their lips, clear their throat, hum, laugh, or fiddle with their clothes. Often they seem to stare at something. These actions are purposeless, and people often look like they are behaving strangely during a seizure. Although complex partial seizures can look different in different people, each person tends to carry out the same actions every time they have a seizure. Someone who clears his or her throat and fiddles with his or her clothes is likely to repeat this behavior in their seizures. Complex partial seizures last between 1 and 10 minutes. There is no treatment that would reliably stop these seizures more quickly.

Some people experience a warning (also called an "aura"), which tells them they are going to have a seizure. After the seizure, people may feel tired or confused for a while and may not feel normal for hours.

Around one in three people with epilepsy has complex partial seizures. This type of seizure can affect anyone. Sometimes, complex partial seizures cannot be stopped with antiepileptic drugs. In this case, epilepsy surgery can be considered. It is often unclear what has caused complex partial seizures. Recent research shows how complicated the development of epilepsy can be. It was noted that adults who had "complicated febrile seizures" in childhood have a higher risk of developing epilepsy with complex partial seizures in later life.

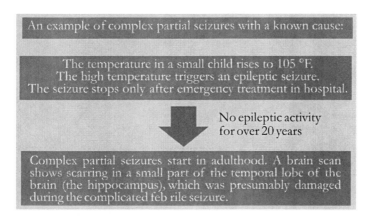

An example of complex partial seizures with a known cause:

The temperature in a small child rises to 105 °F. The high temperature triggers an epileptic seizure. The seizure stops only after emergency treatment in hospital.

No epileptic activity for over 20 years

Complex partial seizures start in adulthood. A brain scan shows scarring in a small part of the temporal lobe of the brain (the hippocampus), which was presumably damaged during the complicated feb rile seizure.

Example

Mrs. K.'s seizures begin with a warning. She knows that she is going to have a seizure and usually sits down. Then her face seems to express a mixture of surprise and distress. During the seizure she may look at someone when her name is called but she never answers. She just stares and makes odd movements with her mouth, as if she was tasting something. Sometimes she grabs the arm of a chair and squeezes it. If she has two seizures in the same day, they make her tired, so she often goes to sleep after the second one.

PARTIAL SEIZURE: SIMPLE OR COMPLEX WITH SECONDARY GENERALIZATION

A partial seizure starts from one area in the surface layer of the brain. In a "simple partial seizure" consciousness is not affected, but in a "complex partial seizure" consciousness is reduced or lost. If the epileptic activity causing partial seizures spreads and involves the whole brain, a tonic-clonic seizure occurs. During a tonic-clonic seizure, the whole body stiffens and shakes. This kind of seizure may be frightening to see unless someone knows what to do. Tonic-clonic seizures are potentially dangerous because they can cause people to fall to the ground with little warning and to injure themselves.

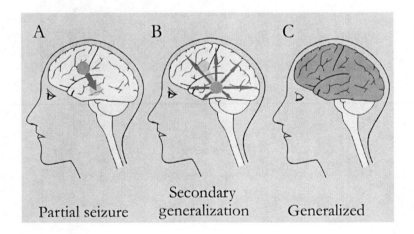

Partial seizure   Secondary generalization   Generalized

It is not completely clear what happens when epileptic activity spreads from one area to the whole brain. This process is called "secondary generalization". The pictures illustrate the spread of epileptic activity. The epileptic activity around the focus, where seizures start, marked by a dot in (A), may only cause twitching of the muscles in the face, for example. However, the epileptic activity also affects other parts of the brain (B), which may then cause spread of the epileptic activity to the whole brain (C).

A single epileptic seizure does not damage the brain. However, seizures can cause injuries if they lead to falls or other accidents. Very occasionally, one seizure can also lead to another, without allowing the person to recover in between. This is called "status epilepticus" and is a medical emergency. Status epilepticus can develop from all types of seizures: simple partial, complex partial, and secondary generalized seizures.

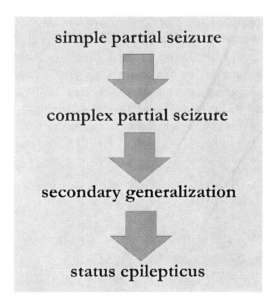

Usually, partial seizures stop without causing spread of epileptic activity throughout the brain. If generalization occurs, it typically causes a single generalized tonic-clonic seizure. Status epilepticus is comparatively rare.

The best choice of antiepileptic drug treatment depends on whether tonic-clonic seizures are caused by epileptic activity that involves the whole brain from the start of a seizure (primary generalized) or whether epileptic activity starts in one part, or focus, of the brain (secondary generalized). For instance, epilepsy surgery may be a treatment option for secondary generalized but not for primary generalized seizures. On the other hand, some antiepileptic drugs work better in primary than in secondary generalized seizures.

The words "partial" and "generalized" do not say how serious, frightening, disabling, or severe different seizures can be. While some partial seizures are very unpleasant and cannot be stopped easily with drugs, some generalized seizures respond readily to medication.

AURA: A PARTIAL SEIZURE THAT CANNOT BE SEEN BY OTHERS

In a partial seizure, epileptic activity only affects one part of the brain. Often, other people do not notice a partial seizure. The person having the seizure may feel, hear, or see things that are not actually there, as if they had imagined them. Such sensations are called "auras." If the epileptic activity causing an aura spreads to an area of the brain that deals with movement, behavior, or consciousness, other people will be able to notice it. People describe many different types of auras. Auras may consist of a tingling feeling in one arm, seeing lights, or being aware of a funny taste. An aura is felt at the very beginning of an epileptic seizure (but many people with epilepsy never have an aura that they can remember after the seizure).

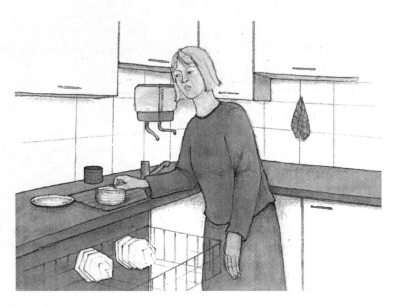

Loading dishes

The young woman in the picture has just come home from a busy day at work. She is loading up her dishwasher. The stress of the day is over and she is beginning to relax a little. In some people, seizures mostly occur when they are winding down after a stressful period.

If people have an aura before a visible seizure, they can use the warning it gives them. They may go somewhere where they can be on their own if they do not want others to see their seizures, or they can sit down to stop themselves from falling over. Some people have learned to control their brain activity so that an aura does not turn into a bigger seizure. They may try to think of a certain smell, bring back a pleasant memory, or rub their forearms, for example. Usually, it is a matter of trial and error to find out whether anything can stop a bigger seizure from developing.

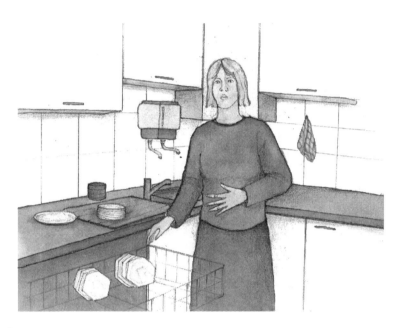

During an aura

The picture shows the young woman pressing her hand on her stomach. She has an odd sensation there and knows that she is going to have a bigger seizure. She has noticed that she can sometimes stop the seizure by concentrating on a particular song. However, this does not always work.

LONG SEIZURES—STATUS EPILEPTICUS

The condition where one seizure is quickly followed by another is called "status epilepticus" ("epileptic state"). Any seizure can develop into status epilepticus. For instance, there is tonic-clonic status, absence status, and complex partial status. Tonic-clonic status is a medical emergency and has to be treated immediately.

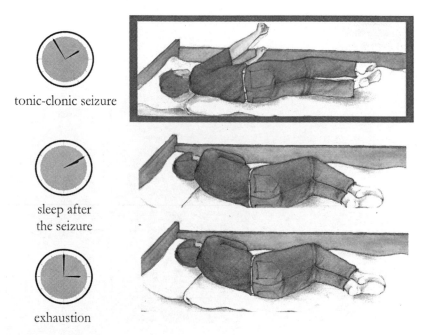

tonic-clonic seizure

sleep after
the seizure

exhaustion

A single tonic-clonic seizure

This picture shows a single tonic-clonic seizure, which lasts about 1 minute. Fifteen minutes later, the man is asleep. After 1 hour, he wakes up. He feels tired and worn out, has a headache, and has bitten the edge of his tongue. A single tonic-clonic seizure does not usually need emergency treatment. There may of course be exceptions to this, for instance, if someone has fallen and was injured during the seizure.

The picture below shows tonic-clonic status epilepticus. This is a medical emergency. Tonic-clonic seizures that go on for longer than 5 minutes or that happen again after a short break have to be treated immediately, and an ambulance should be called.

Tonic-clonic status is dangerous because it stops normal breathing so that the brain does not get enough oxygen. It becomes more dangerous the longer it lasts. Status epilepticus can be stopped with medication more than 9 out of 10 times. If tonic-clonic status lasts for over 1 hour, there is about a 10% risk of death, even if the person is cared for in an intensive care unit. That's why it is so important to seek medical treatment immediately.

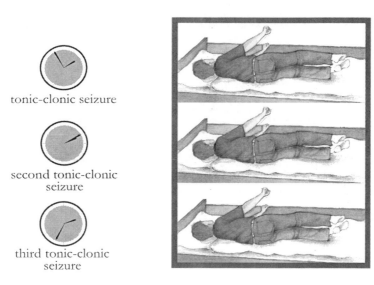

tonic-clonic seizure

second tonic-clonic
seizure

third tonic-clonic
seizure

Status epilepticus

Some types of status epilepticus are difficult to recognize. People in absence or complex partial status, for example, may simply seem confused or slow. Such types are also known as "non-convulsive status epilepticus" because they do not cause shaking or jerking of muscles. People in non-convulsive status may be able to do simple things like feed themselves or get dressed. If examined carefully, their eyelids sometimes twitch slightly. However, it takes an EEG to confirm that someone is in non-convulsive status epilepticus.

MOST PEOPLE WITH EPILEPSY HAVE SEIZURES OF ONE TYPE

The classification of seizures and of epilepsy is important because it can help people to get the best treatment. For instance, if the diagnosis is childhood absence epilepsy, drugs can be stopped after a few years because seizures are likely to have disappeared.

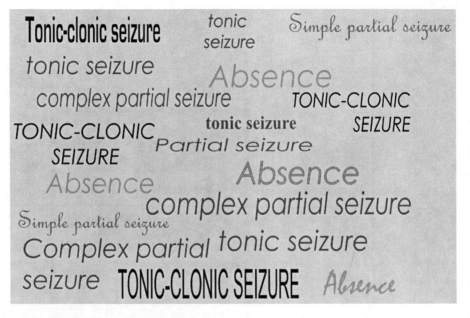

The different types of print in this picture can be grouped together based on the size and shape of the letter.

The first step in the classification of seizures is to recognize the type of seizure. Is it focal or generalized? The next step is to try to identify an epileptic syndrome on the basis of the range of the observed seizure types. Sometimes it is impossible to classify seizures or an epilepsy syndrome.

In one person, all seizures tend to be similar.

1.3 EPILEPSIES ARE DIVIDED INTO SYNDROMES

EPILEPSY SYNDROMES ARE NAMES FOR DIFFERENT TYPES OF EPILEPSY

Apart from the classification of epileptic seizures, there is a classification of epilepsy syndromes. These syndromes have been discovered and described over the last 200 years.

There are many features that distinguish different types of epilepsy, for instance the age at the onset of seizures, or the particular seizure types. These features were described in people who had epilepsy in the past. They allow experts to divide epilepsy into different epilepsy syndromes. There are typical features for each syndrome.

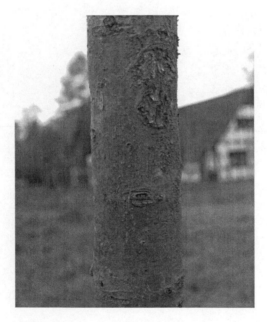

"Syndromes" are recognized in all areas of life. When a gardener discovers a particular type of mark on the bark of a fruit tree and notices that the leaves of this tree are turning brown, he knows that these changes are caused by a particular type of beetle. He can find out from other gardeners how they have dealt with this particular beetle in the past.

It makes sense to split epilepsy into different syndromes because recognizing these syndromes gives us information about whether seizures are likely to stop or not and about the kind of treatment that is most likely to help. For instance, a drug may have helped other people with a particular epilepsy syndrome in the past; it is likely that this drug will work in the same syndrome now. In some syndromes, epileptic activity stops at a particular age. In other syndromes, medication has to be taken for life. Knowing the name of their epilepsy syndrome allows people to understand a little better what the future may hold for them.

Being diagnosed with a particular epilepsy syndrome only means that it is likely that the epileptic seizures will respond to treatment in a particular way. There is no certainty that this will actually happen. For instance, epileptic seizures may continue, although they usually stop at a certain age in the particular epilepsy syndrome. There may be no explanation for such unexpected developments.

The list shows which features can make up an epilepsy syndrome

The age at which the seizures begin

The type or types of seizures

The cause of the seizures

The part of the brain involved

Factors that provoke seizures

How severe and how frequent seizures are

The relationship of seizures to sleep

Certain patterns in the EEG

Other symptoms (in addition to seizures)

The prospect of recovery

Not every syndrome is defined by all of these features. One of the oldest epilepsy syndromes, which was recognized by specialists, was a form of epilepsy that the doctor W. J. West observed in his son. Dr. West's description has enabled other doctors to recognize his son's epilepsy syndrome in other people. This particular type of epilepsy is now called "West syndrome."

EPILEPSY SYNDROMES IN BABIES: INFANTILE SPASMS, BENIGN NEONATAL CONVULSIONS

Epileptic seizures in babies look different from those in older children or adults because the baby's brain is not fully developed. There are seizure types and epilepsy syndromes that are only seen in this age group.

Infantile spasms (West syndrome)

The seizures begin between 3 and 18 months of age. They consist of sudden jerks or "infantile spasms." The baby suddenly throws his arms up and brings his head and chest forward. Infantile spasms are sometimes called "jack-knife" seizures because they cause the baby to suddenly fold up like a jackknife. Another seizure type that may be seen in West syndrome is a tonic seizure, which can last a little longer. During a tonic seizure, the arms may be raised and stretched out. Seizures occur most commonly just after waking up.

Babies with this epilepsy syndrome seem to stop developing and may lose skills that they had already mastered, such as sitting, rolling over, or babbling. In most cases, West syndrome is caused by brain disorders or injuries. Sometimes no cause can be found. The EEG shows an unusual pattern called *hypsarrhythmia*, even in between seizures. This is a very irregular pattern that helps to confirm the diagnosis. Over the longer term, most children with infantile spasms will develop learning difficulties, especially those children whose spasms are related to a brain disorder or injury. The outlook is better for children who were developing well before the spasms started. A small number of children develop normally once the seizures have stopped. Many experts believe that it is important for children's long-term development to stop seizures quickly. Some children with infantile spasms later develop other kinds of epilepsy, for instance Lennox-Gastaut syndrome. They may also develop autism or other learning difficulties.

Two months ago, this boy's mother noticed that he was having brief periodic spasms of his body. While he is being filmed in the hospital, his blanket has been removed so that the movements can be seen better. Often there are several spasms in a row, called serial seizures. Sometimes he cries when they are over. Seizures in babies can look very similar to normal movements, so they are sometimes difficult to spot.

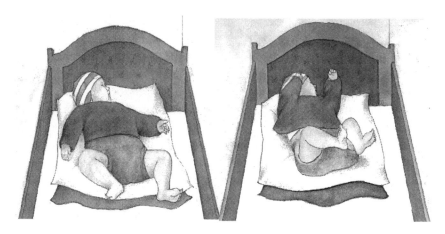

Resting   During a seizure

Benign neonatal convulsions

These seizures are called "benign" because most children recover without developing epilepsy or learning difficulties in later life. The seizures begin in the first week of life. The seizures consist of sudden jerks or short pauses in the normal breathing pattern. They can occur several times during the day. Seizures usually stop without treatment. The further development of children is normal, and there is no risk of developing a different type of epilepsy later in life. Sometimes benign convulsions run in the family. In those cases, there is a slightly increased risk of developing a different type of epilepsy later in life.

EPILEPSY SYNDROMES IN CHILDHOOD: LENNOX-GASTAUT SYNDROME

Lennox-Gastaut syndrome (LGS) is a severe form of childhood epilepsy with frequent seizures of many different types. The seizures begin between 1 and 8 years of age. There are different types of seizures. Atonic seizures cause sudden episodes of loss of muscle tone that cause the child to fall to the ground. Absences are short episodes when the child goes blank and seems to stare. Tonic seizures last about 10–20 seconds and consist of stiffening of the arms or legs, and the eyes may roll up. Myoclonic seizures cause brief twitches of limbs or trunk. There are also tonic-clonic seizures, which cause the body and limbs to stiffen and jerk. LGS can have different causes. Possible causes include inflammation of the brain, lack of oxygen during birth, abnormal development of the brain while still in the womb, or metabolic disorders. Sometimes no cause is found.

The EEG of children with LGS often shows irregular slow activity even when there is no obvious seizure. EEG abnormalities can be seen most clearly during sleep. The EEG changes of LGS are so clear that EEG is helpful in finding out whether or not a child suffers from this syndrome. The long-term outcome is often poor. In some children no antiepileptic drug seems to work. Others need more than one drug for seizure control. Sometimes seizures cannot be stopped completely, and medication only reduces the number or severity of seizures. Most children with LGS continue to have seizures and develop a degree of learning difficulties.

Epilepsy syndromes in childhood: Childhood absence epilepsy

Childhood absence epilepsy (CAE) is a mild form of epilepsy that typically goes away during teenage years. The seizures begin between 4 and 8 years of age. The seizures consist of staring spells during which the child is not responsive. Each spell lasts about 10 seconds and starts and stops abruptly. The child is not aware that anything has happened. These seizures can occur many times per day. Some children with CAE develop tonic-clonic seizures. In these seizures, the whole body stiffens and jerks.

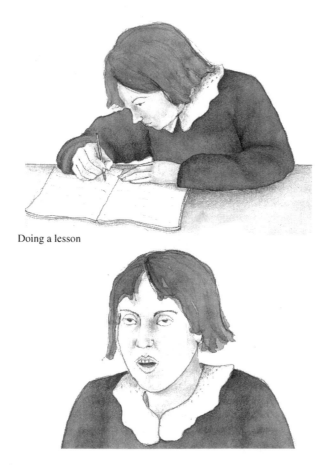

Doing a lesson

During a seizure

The cause of CAE is unknown. Sometimes this form of epilepsy runs in the family. The EEG shows very typical changes during absence seizures. The outlook is good because seizures usually respond to treatment and disappear in 2 out of 3 children during adolescence.

EPILEPSY SYNDROMES IN CHILDHOOD: LANDAU-KLEFFNER SYNDROME, RASMUSSEN'S SYNDROME

Landau-Kleffner syndrome

Landau-Kleffner syndrome (LKS) is a rare disorder in which seizures occur together with speech problems. The seizures begin between 3 and 7 years of age. The speech disorder may start suddenly or slowly. It usually affects the understanding of speech but can also affect speaking. Children with LKS usually have tonic-clonic seizures, in which the body and limbs stiffen and jerk, and absences (staring spells). The cause of LKS is unknown. Sometimes LKS runs in families. The EEG shows very typical changes, especially during sleep, so sleep recordings are very important. The seizures stop in 4 out of 5 children after the age of 10. Seizures can usually be stopped before this age with antiepileptic drugs. However, these drugs do not help for the speech problems, which can persist long term.

Rasmussen's syndrome

Rasmussen's syndrome is a progressive neurologic disorder. This means that it tends to get worse over time. Seizures are often the first problem to appear. The seizures begin between 1 and 14 years of age. They consist of simple partial motor seizures, for instance, of twitches in one hand. Rasmussen's syndrome often causes status epilepticus of partial motor seizures. In this form of status epilepticus, twitching can continue for hours or days, although consciousness is not lost. Rasmussen's syndrome tends to affect only one-half of the brain. This means that motor seizures are usually limited to one side of the body. The syndrome is thought to be caused by an overactivity of the body's immune system. The process may be triggered by a viral infection. A blood test may be helpful in recognizing the infection. The outlook for seizure control is often poor. It may be impossible to stop seizures, and the body part affected by the seizures may become weak or even paralyzed. On the other hand, the condition may also stop getting worse. The treatment may not only consist of drugs to stop seizures but also medication to reduce the activity of the body's immune system or brain surgery.

Epilepsy syndromes in Childhood: Benign Rolandic epilepsy

Rolandic epilepsy (benign partial epilepsy of childhood with centro-temporal spikes) is a particularly common type of epilepsy in childhood that does not need to be treated in most cases.

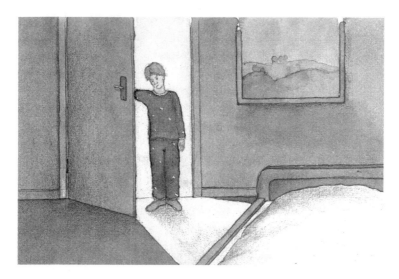

This child was woken up by a seizure in the early hours of the morning and has run to his parents' bedroom. The right half of the face tenses up during seizures.

Rolandic epilepsy usually begins between the ages of 3 and 13 (mostly between 6 and 8 years of age). The seizures cause twitching, numbness, or tingling of the child's face or tongue. Seizures often happen in sleep and can cause the children to produce gurgling or retching noises. Seizures last no longer than 2 minutes and usually do not affect consciousness. Sometimes children with Rolandic epilepsy have tonic-clonic seizures (in which the body and limbs stiffen and jerk). These seizures typically occur during sleep. Antiepileptic drugs are usually very effective if they are needed.

The cause of Rolandic epilepsy is unknown. Sometimes this form of epilepsy runs in families. The EEG shows very typical changes. The outlook is good. Seizures usually stop on their own by the age of 15.

EPILEPSY SYNDROMES IN TEENS: JUVENILE MYOCLONIC EPILEPSY, JUVENILE ABSENCE EPILEPSY

Juvenile myoclonic epilepsy

Juvenile myoclonic epilepsy (JME) is a common form of epilepsy that sometimes runs in families. Seizures begin between 8 and 18 years of age. There are different types of seizures in JME. Myoclonic seizures cause brief jerks of the arms, shoulders, or occasionally the legs. Jerks can occur in a series and are sometimes followed by tonic-clonic seizures (which cause the body and limbs to stiffen and jerk). In absence seizures, people stop and stare for several seconds. Some people with JME notice that their seizures are triggered by flickering lights, such as strobe lights in nightclubs, TV sets, video games, or light shining through trees or bouncing off ocean waves or snow. People who experience this are said to have "photosensitive" seizures. Occasionally, myoclonic seizures can also be triggered by making decisions or by doing mental arithmetic.

The cause of JME is unknown. Several factors can bring on seizures in JME, such as lack of sleep, stress, and alcohol. Seizures tend to occur in the early morning, after a nap, or during the night. Some children with childhood absence epilepsy later develop JME. The EEG often shows typical changes, especially in people with photosensitive seizures. The outlook for people with JME is good. The seizures can usually be controlled with antiepileptic drugs. However, treatment typically has to be taken for life. When antiepileptic medication is stopped, seizures reappear in 9 out of 10 people. Even people who have been seizure-free for years usually have seizures again if they stop taking their medication. People with JME have the same intellectual ability as other people in general.

Juvenile absence epilepsy

Juvenile absence epilepsy (JAE) is relatively common. The seizures begin between the ages of 8 and 18. They consist of absences (staring spells), which may occur many times per day. Additional tonic-clonic seizures (which cause the body and limbs to stiffen and shake) occur in 1 out of 5 people with this form of epilepsy. Some people with JAE do not realize they are having seizures until they have had a tonic-clonic seizure. The seizures often occur shortly after awakening but they can happen at other times during the day.

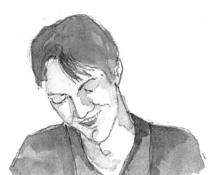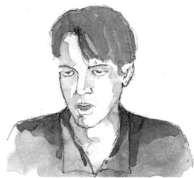

The picture on the left shows a young man during a conversation. He suddenly stops talking and has an absence attack. The picture on the right shows his empty look during the attack. He stares ahead for about 5 seconds, his eyelids twitch a little, and the attack is over after a few more seconds. He does not know that he has had a seizure, although he sometimes realizes that there is a brief gap in his memory.

The cause of JAE is not known, but it is felt to be similar to CAE. Sometimes JAE runs in families. There is a good chance of controlling seizures fully in this epileptic syndrome. However, most persons with JAE need to continue to take medication for life. To maintain seizure control, they may also need to avoid a lack of sleep and abstain from alcohol or use it only moderately.

EPILEPSY SYNDROMES IN TEENS: PROGRESSIVE MYOCLONUS EPILEPSY

Progressive myoclonic epilepsies

This is a group of rare disorders in which people have myoclonic (brief jerks) and tonic-clonic seizures (the body stiffens and shakes). Most of these disorders also cause other problems like unsteadiness, stiffness of the limbs, and mental deterioration. Tests can identify the cause of most of these disorders.

MELAS

Mitochondrial, encephalopathy, lactic acidosis, and stroke-like episodes (MELAS) is a rare disorder in which mitochondria do not work properly. Mitochondria can be found in all cells of the body. They produce energy for the cells. People with MELAS can have both generalized and partial seizures. They can also have strokes at a young age.

Myoclonus epilepsy with ragged red fibers (MERRF)

This is another disorder caused by a problem with the body's mitochondria. People with MERRF have tonic-clonic and myoclonic seizures. It can also be associated with hearing loss and dementia.

Baltic myoclonus (Unverricht-Lundborg disease)

Baltic myoclonus begins between 6 and 15 years of age. It is an inherited disease that occurs particularly in the Baltic region, Southern Europe, and North Africa. People develop sudden jerks (myoclonic seizures), which can be triggered by stimulation, and tonic-clonic seizures. Baltic myoclonus also causes loss of other brain functions and gets worse with time.

Lafora body disease

In this disease, several organs are affected: brain, heart, muscles, liver, and others. In addition to myoclonic seizures, people may develop tonic-clonic seizures. Other symptoms include dementia and visual loss.

EPILEPSY SYNDROMES IN TEENS: EPILEPSY WITH TONIC-CLONIC SEIZURES ON AWAKENING

These are tonic-clonic seizures that occur shortly after waking up. The seizures begin between the ages of 10 and 25. In these seizures, the body and limbs stiffen and shake. Seizures only happen within 2 hours of waking up. This is so typical that most people with this epilepsy syndrome know that they will not have a seizure more than 2 hours after waking up. Sometimes they also have seizures with a short interruption of consciousness (absences) or brief jerks (myoclonic seizures).

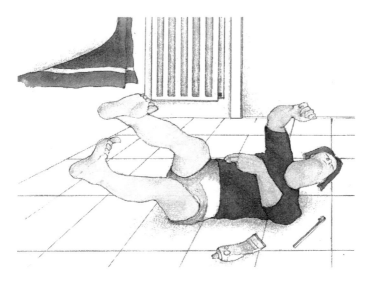

The picture shows a young man having a tonic-clonic seizure in the bathroom

The EEG often shows typical changes, even in between seizures. Seizures are more likely if people have not had enough sleep. This is called "sleep deprivation." This shows that sleep is very important for people with this type of epilepsy. Sleeping long enough and sleeping regularly can help to stop seizures. The cause of this epilepsy syndrome is not known. Seizures can usually be stopped easily with antiepileptic drugs. However, most people with tonic-clonic seizures on awakening need to take medication for life.

TEMPORAL LOBE EPILEPSY

The major parts of the brain consist of two halves, the left and right hemispheres. The hemispheres are divided into four "lobes." The temporal lobe is marked in the picture. This lobe is particularly important for feelings, emotions, and memory.

Partial seizures often start in the temporal lobes. Temporal lobe epilepsy can start at any age. Sometimes it develops after a head injury or an infection such as meningitis. Often the cause is unknown.

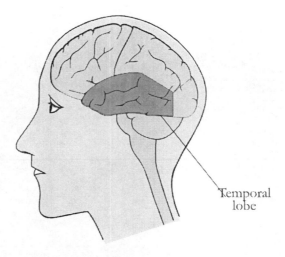

Temporal lobe

The "hippocampus" and "amygdala" are on the inside of the temporal lobes. They are important for learning, memory, and emotions such as fear.

Seizures from the temporal lobes often begin with a warning (aura). This can last several seconds or longer. During an aura, people may experience feelings, emotions, or thoughts that appear very familiar or completely alien to them. Auras are often difficult to describe. People may also be aware of a sensation rising up from their stomach or they may hear voices or experience an odd taste or smell. Following this, they become unresponsive or they respond oddly when spoken to. People may carry out strange actions like lip smacking, rubbing their hands together, laughing, shouting, or fiddling with buttons or clothes.

Often people stare at something and cannot be distracted from it. The seizure stops after 1–5 minutes but people remain confused or tired afterward. Some people complain of a headache.

In 3 out of 5 people with temporal lobe epilepsy, seizures sometimes spread from the temporal lobe to both hemispheres of the brain (secondary generalization). The result is a tonic-clonic seizure in which the body and limbs stiffen and shake.

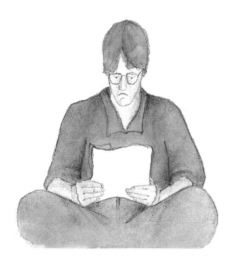

Reading

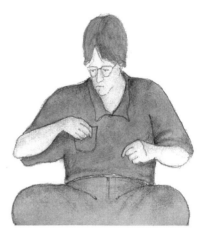

During a seizure in the temporal lobe

Unfortunately, antiepileptic drugs stop seizures in only 3 out of 5 people with temporal lobe epilepsy, even when different drugs and combinations of drugs have been tried. It is not known why some people with temporal lobe epilepsy respond to medication and others do not.

If drugs have been tried without success, then other treatments may be considered. Some people with temporal lobe epilepsy can benefit from epilepsy surgery. This involves an operation in which the part of the temporal lobe causing the seizures is removed.

FRONTAL LOBE EPILEPSY

The parts of the brain directly behind the forehead and above the eyes are the right and left frontal lobes. In the picture, the left frontal lobe is shaded.

Seizures usually start in a small area of the frontal lobes (partial seizure). In a simple partial seizure, consciousness is not affected, whereas in complex partial seizures, alertness and awareness are reduced or lost. Compared to complex partial seizures starting in the temporal lobe, frontal lobe seizures are shorter and more abrupt in the way they start and stop. Often seizures are more frequent. Frontal lobe seizures have a tendency to happen while sleeping.

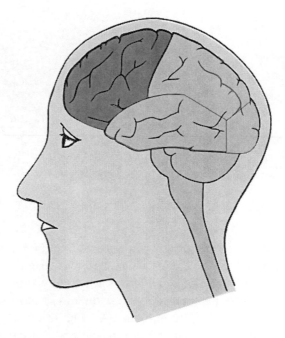

The frontal lobes are important for planning and carrying out movements. They also play a role in motivation and the control of emotions such as anger.

In some people, frontal lobe seizures start with a warning (aura), which is often no more than a feeling that a seizure is going to happen. Frontal lobe seizures can involve laughing, shouting, or crying. In other people, seizures cause weakness or the inability to use certain muscles, such as the muscles that enable someone to speak. Sometimes people remain fully aware while their arms and legs move without their control. Frontal lobe seizures can look so strange to other people that they may be mistaken as emotional or psychological (sometimes called "non-epileptic seizures"). EEG recordings may not help to tell the difference between frontal lobe and non-epileptic seizures because the EEG electrodes can fail to pick up the epileptic discharges in frontal lobe epilepsy.

Although there are many different types of frontal lobe seizures, all seizures in one person tend to be very similar. For instance, a person who moves his legs as if he were peddling on a bicycle during a seizure will move in the same way during other seizures.

The young woman is sitting in a waiting room. She is a little tired. Suddenly she becomes restless and goes into a seizure. There are forceful movements affecting the whole body. She is fully aware during the seizure but she cannot stop the movements although she has injured herself badly in her seizures before.

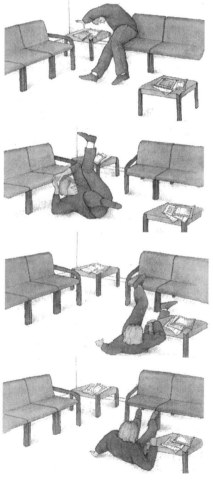

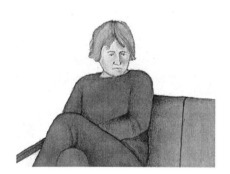

Sitting

Sometimes frontal lobe seizures cannot be controlled with medication. If antiepileptic drugs are not effective, vagus nerve stimulation or epilepsy surgery may help. However, seizures starting in the frontal lobe are harder to stop with surgery than temporal lobe seizures.

During a seizure

PARIETAL LOBE EPILEPSY

The parietal lobes are behind the frontal lobes and above the temporal lobes. The left parietal lobe is shaded in the picture.

Seizures starting in the parietal lobes are relatively rare. Epileptic activity may be limited to a small part of the parietal lobe and cause seizures without loss of awareness (simple partial seizure), or it may involve larger parts of the brain and affect alertness and awareness, causing complex partial seizures. As in all partial seizures, epileptic activity can spread to the rest of the brain and cause generalized tonic-clonic seizures in which the body and limbs stiffen and shake. Parietal lobe seizures typically cause sensations in the skin. People may become aware of numbness, tickling, or (very rarely) pain. The sensation may spread from a small area of the body (like one finger) to a larger area (like the hand or arm). This sort of spreading sensation is also called *Jacksonian march* or seizure, named after the famous neurologist of the nineteenth century, Hughlings Jackson.

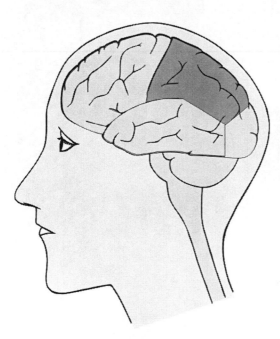

Like other partial seizures, parietal lobe seizures can be caused by abnormalities of the structure of the brain. Such abnormalities may be related to problems with brain development while still in the womb, brain injuries, or brain tumors. However, often brain scans in people with parietal lobe seizures are completely normal. If an abnormality is seen on a scan it can sometimes be removed. Surgery may stop the seizures.

The parietal lobes help to make sense of perceptions from the skin and from the limbs. They also deal with understanding language and reading.

OCCIPITAL LOBE EPILEPSY

The occipital lobes are found at the back of the brain. The left occipital lobe is shaded in the picture.

Partial seizures from the occipital lobes can cause visual symptoms like flashes of light, color, and patterns. People can see more complicated images like faces, people, or scenes from the past if seizures start from the part of the occipital lobes bordering on the parietal or temporal lobes. Seizures may cause temporary blindness. Partial seizures can turn into generalized tonic-clonic seizures in which the body and limbs stiffen and shake.

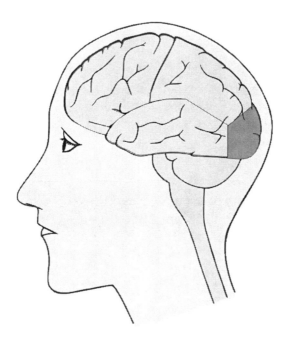

The occipital lobes help the brain to understand the visual information from the eyes.

Seizures from the occipital lobe can spread to the temporal lobe or frontal lobe. If this happens, the symptoms of occipital lobe seizures can be combined with the symptoms of temporal or frontal lobe seizures. This can make occipital lobe seizures hard to recognize.

Occipital lobe seizures can be related to structural abnormalities of the brain. Abnormalities may result from an accident, inflammation, disturbances of blood supply, or tumors. The cause of occipital lobe epilepsy remains unknown in 1 out of 4 people.

EPILEPSY CAUSED BY HEAD TRAUMA, INFLAMMATION, FEVER

A person who has had a severe head injury may have a brief seizure at the time of the injury or during the first week afterwards. Such seizures soon after a head injury often stop without long-term treatment. However, it is more serious if seizures develop later. The risk of developing seizures after a head injury is greatest from 3 months to 3 years after the injury. In rare instances, they can start many years later.

Head trauma

Head injuries cause epilepsy (post-traumatic epilepsy) only in a minority of people. Factors that increase the risk of developing post-traumatic epilepsy are:

- wounds exposing the brain (gun shot, depressed skull fracture)
- injuries that cause bleeding into the brain
- prolonged period of unconsciousness after the injury (longer than 30 minutes)

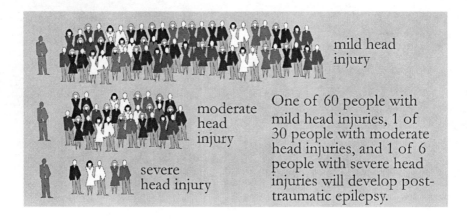

mild head injury

moderate head injury

severe head injury

One of 60 people with mild head injuries, 1 of 30 people with moderate head injuries, and 1 of 6 people with severe head injuries will develop post-traumatic epilepsy.

What happens during a seizure caused by a head injury depends on the location of the injury. For instance, an injury in the front part of the brain (frontal lobe) often leads to seizures that affect alertness and awareness, and that cause shaking of the muscles. Injuries of the temporal lobes can lead to seizures during which people experience odd smells, ideas, or sounds.

Inflammation

To remain healthy, the human body constantly has to fight off viruses, bacteria, and other small organisms. The brain is quite well protected against injury to the skull and its lining, but sometimes infections overcome these barriers. An infection of the brain (encephalitis) or of its lining (meningitis) may be life-threatening. In addition, 1 out of 17 people with encephalitis or meningitis develop epilepsy later.

Fever

Between the ages of 3 months and 5 years, children may develop seizures when they have a high temperature, even if there is no infection of the brain. These seizures are called *febrile seizures*.

Simple febrile seizures are single seizures lasting less than 15 minutes. They occur in otherwise healthy children and are rarely associated with any brain abnormality. The risk of epilepsy in later life is only slightly increased. In most cases, children do not need to stay in the hospital or take antiepileptic medication.

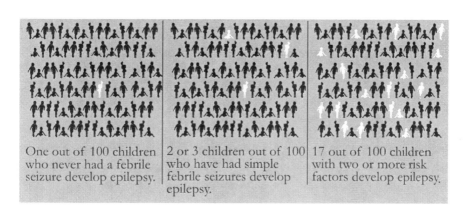

One out of 100 children who never had a febrile seizure develop epilepsy. | 2 or 3 children out of 100 who have had simple febrile seizures develop epilepsy. | 17 out of 100 children with two or more risk factors develop epilepsy.

Complex febrile seizures also occur with fever and without infection of the brain. A febrile seizure is called complex if (1) it lasted longer than 15 minutes, (2) it was a partial seizure, (3) there was more than one seizure in 24 hours, or (4) the child is left with a neurological problem (such as weakness after the seizure). If two or more of these risk factors apply, there is a higher risk of developing epilepsy later in life.

There is no evidence that antiepileptic medication can prevent the development of epilepsy after complex febrile seizures.

EPILEPSY ASSOCIATED WITH MULTIPLE SCLEROSIS

Multiple sclerosis (MS) is a chronic disorder of the nervous system. This means that it does not go away once it has started. About 1 in 15 people develop epileptic seizures at some time during the illness. On average, seizures begin 7 years after the onset of MS. The seizures usually start in a small area (partial seizures, e.g. brief jerks), but seizures can generalize (secondary generalized seizures, in which the body and limbs stiffen and shake). People with MS can also develop painful tonic spasms in which limbs get stiff. These can sometimes be blocked with antiepileptic drugs although they are not caused by epileptic discharges in the brain.

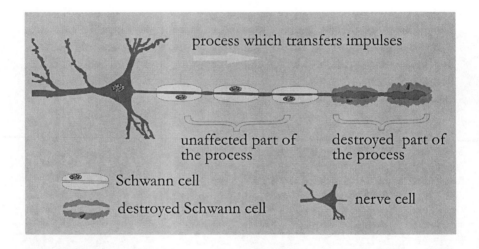

Nerve cells are connected to processes that look a bit like the tentacles of an octopus and that start in the body of one nerve cell. Nerve cells "talk" to each other by sending electric impulses along these processes. Different types of cells (Schwann cells) insulate the processes so that they can carry electric impulses more efficiently. In MS, this insulation is attacked by the body's immune system. Sometimes this sort of damage causes epileptic activity. The body can repair the damage to the insulation of the nerve process to some extent. However, the repair is usually not perfect, which means that people with MS often develop more symptoms as they get older.

1.4 SEIZURES BRIEFLY INTERRUPT THE NORMAL WORKING OF THE BRAIN

EPILEPTIC SEIZURES COME FROM THE BRAIN, AND THEY INTERRUPT NORMAL BRAIN FUNCTION

What form a seizure takes depends on the part of the brain it comes from. In the movement areas of the brain, for instance, each area of brain deals with the movements of one particular part of the body. Brain areas are linked to the muscles by nerves. If one part of the movement area of the brain is damaged and produces epileptic discharges, jerking may be seen in the muscles that are controlled by the affected part of the brain.

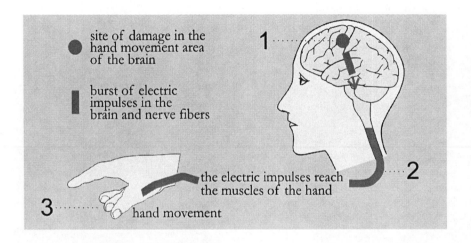

site of damage in the hand movement area of the brain

1

burst of electric impulses in the brain and nerve fibers

the electric impulses reach the muscles of the hand

2

3   hand movement

The picture gives an example. A small part of the brain (1), marked by the dot, is damaged. Epileptic activity is produced in this damaged area. The episode (or burst) of epileptic activity runs through the nerves to the thumb (2). The thumb twitches every time a burst of electric impulses from the brain reaches the muscles in the hand (3). If the place in the brain where the impulses come from shifts a little, or if it grows and a greater area of the brain starts to send out epileptic activity, the jerking can affect other parts of the hand or the whole hand, or other types of symptoms not involving muscle movements may occur. Bursts of electric impulses are typical of epileptic activity.

> The appearance of a seizure can show where it comes from in the brain.

THE BRAIN IS DIVIDED INTO SEVERAL PARTS

Each half of the brain (or "hemisphere") is divided into four "lobes." They are marked in the picture.

The frontal lobes

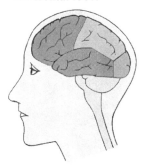

The frontal lobes are important for the planning and control of movements. "Hypermotor" and "Jacksonian seizures" start in the frontal lobes.

The parietal lobes

The parietal lobes deal with sensation. Relatively few epileptic seizures start in the parietal lobes. One example is a focal seizure in which people feel an odd sensation spreading over their body.

The temporal lobes

The temporal lobes contain the "hippocampus," the "amygdala," and the hearing centers of the brain. The hippocampus is important for learning and memory, and the amygdala for emotions. Both are common starting points of epileptic seizures. They can sometimes be removed with surgery to stop epilepsy.

The occipital lobes

The occipital lobes contain the centers of the brain, which allow us to see. Seizures rarely come from this lobe. If they do, they can cause people to see flashes of lights.

ALL MOVEMENTS ARE CONTROLLED BY THE BRAIN

Different parts of the brain work together to control movements. One particularly important area is marked in the picture. The centers of the brain that plan more complicated movements are in front of this area.

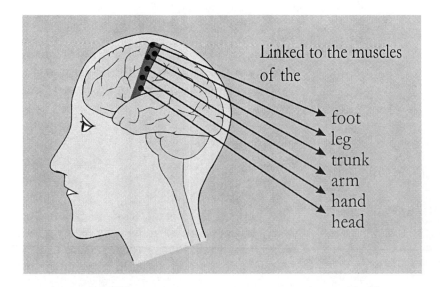

Linked to the muscles of the

foot
leg
trunk
arm
hand
head

The area marked is linked to all muscles of the body. Parts that are close to each other within this area are linked to neighboring muscle groups. How much space each muscle group takes up in the brain depends on how complicated its movements are. The muscles of the hand, which have to do fine and complicated tasks, and those of the face, which have to produce many different expressions, take up more space than the muscles of the thigh, for example.

Muscles do not work properly if the center that controls them in the brain is damaged.

THE PARTS OF THE BRAIN THAT DIRECT MOVEMENT
CAN PRODUCE CLONIC SEIZURES

These are seizures that consist of muscle twitching that people cannot stop. Which muscles twitch depends on the part of the brain sending out the epileptic activity.

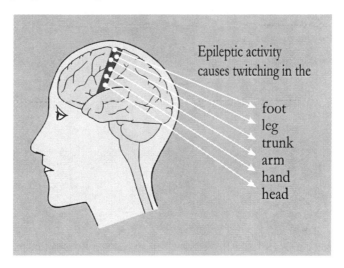

Epileptic activity causes twitching in the

foot
leg
trunk
arm
hand
head

In one person, seizures always start in the same muscles. This shows that the working of the brain is always disturbed in the same place.

Example

When Mr. K. has a seizure, his left thumb twitches about twice in 1 second. After a short while, the twitching spreads. First, there is twitching of all fingers of the left hand, then of the whole hand. Eventually, the forearm starts to jerk, then the whole arm and shoulder. He has Jacksonian seizures, in which epileptic activity spreads gradually over the surface of the brain.

PARTS OF THE BRAIN THAT ARE ACTIVE WHEN PEOPLE FEEL HAPPY, ANXIOUS, OR SAD

The centers of the brain important for emotions are found in the "limbic system."

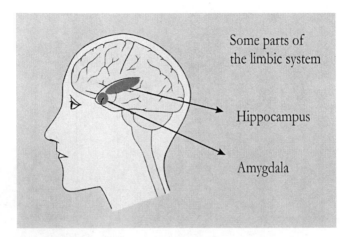

Some parts of the limbic system

Hippocampus

Amygdala

The different parts of the limbic system are deep inside the brain. They are not visible on the surface. The limbic system is found in both hemispheres. This system is sometimes called the "emotional brain." It is also important for memory, however. We do not know exactly how it produces emotions like sadness, joy, or anger. When it is damaged people can have emotional problems. They are more likely to become depressed or anxious and can find it difficult to recognize emotions in other people.

> Damage to the limbic system can cause emotional and memory problems.

PARTIAL SEIZURES CAN START IN THE LIMBIC SYSTEM

Partial seizures from the limbic system often start with a warning (aura) of a "funny sensation" in the stomach or chest. This sensation may rise up into the throat.

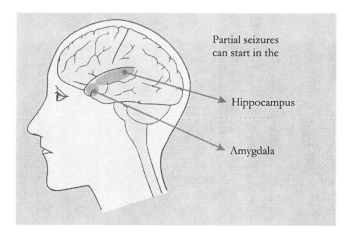

Partial seizures can start in the

Hippocampus

Amygdala

Seizures can also start with loss of awareness. Some important parts of the limbic system are in the temporal lobes. In some people, whose seizures cannot be stopped with antiepileptic drugs, an operation may be possible to remove these parts.

Example

Mrs. P. has noticed that she always has partial seizures when she feels depressed. She has managed to stop seizures by concentrating hard on nice memories from her childhood whenever she gets the odd sensation in her stomach that tells her that a seizure is coming on.

THE WORLD OUTSIDE IS PICTURED IN THE BRAIN

The information picked up by the eyes, ears, and other senses is passed through the nerves to the sensation areas of the brain. The brain centers in these areas enable the brain to put together a picture of the outside world.

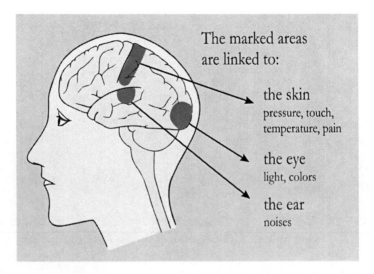

The marked areas are linked to:

the skin
pressure, touch, temperature, pain

the eye
light, colors

the ear
noises

These areas of the brain are like screens onto which sensations from the body surface, the pictures from the eyes, and sounds from the ears are projected. When you draw a letter on your skin, for instance, this letter is projected onto the surface of the brain in the form of electric activity. Seeing a flash of light with your eyes causes a flash of electric activity in the vision center of the brain. If this center was stimulated with electric activity through an electrode placed on the surface of the brain, you would think that you had seen a flash of light, even though no actual flash of light occurred. Likewise, stimulating the hearing centers of the brain would produce the sensation of hearing a noise, and stimulating the skin areas of the brain would cause a feeling of being touched.

SEIZURES FROM THE VISION AREAS OF THE BRAIN PRODUCE IMAGES LIKE IN A DREAM

If epileptic activity does not spread outside the areas that deal with sensation, seizures may only consist of a perception. Such a perception would, of course, only be noticed by the person having the seizure.

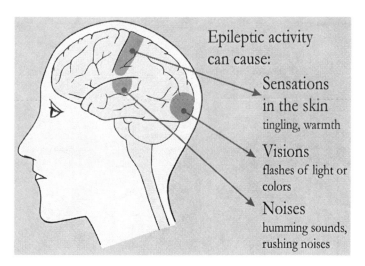

Epileptic activity can cause:

Sensations in the skin
tingling, warmth

Visions
flashes of light or colors

Noises
humming sounds, rushing noises

Epileptic seizures from these areas of the brain are called "sensory seizures." They are partial seizures that can spread and turn into tonic-clonic seizures.

Example

Mrs. L. had attacks of tingling that always affected the same spot on her right arm. She was not aware of any trigger for the tingling. Sometimes there were a series of these feelings. After some time, she had a tonic-clonic seizure after having several episodes of tingling in a row. She had a range of tests and was found to have a brain tumor. The attacks of tingling stopped after the tumor was removed.

THE RETICULAR FORMATION CAN SWITCH ATTENTION ON OR OFF

Hearing or seeing things does not just depend on the hearing or vision centers of the brain alone. The brain also has to switch these centers on. One important part of the brain that is involved in switching on attention and allowing people to focus and concentrate is the "reticular formation."

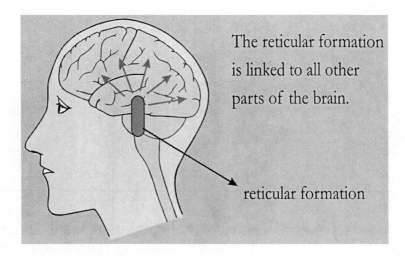

The reticular formation is linked to all other parts of the brain.

reticular formation

People can only see, hear, and feel things if their reticular formation enables them to pay attention to lights, sounds, or sensations. The reticular formation also plays an important role in waking us up in the mornings. People whose reticular formation has been damaged are very sleepy.

Waking up and being awake depends on the reticular formation.

THE RETICULAR FORMATION PLAYS AN IMPORTANT ROLE IN GENERALIZED SEIZURES

Given its close connections to the other parts of the brain, it is easy to imagine how epileptic activity can spread from the reticular formation to both hemispheres. Seizures happen most readily when people are tired. For some people, seizures also start shortly after they have fallen asleep or shortly after waking up.

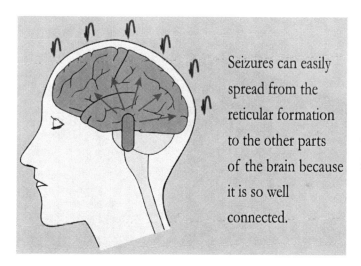

Seizures can easily spread from the reticular formation to the other parts of the brain because it is so well connected.

The picture shows how an absence seizure starts in the reticular formation during light sleep. The EEG shows epileptic spike-and-wave activity over the whole brain.

Example

Mr. D. noticed that his seizures are more likely to strike when he has not slept very much. He now tries to reduce the number of seizures by going to bed and getting up at the same time every day.

EPILEPSY IS OFTEN CAUSED BY A PROBLEM IN ONE SMALL PART OF THE BRAIN

Epileptic seizures stop the affected area of the brain from working normally during the seizure and perhaps for a period of time afterwards. The appearance of seizures from one part of the brain is similar each time. They cause the same movements or perceptions, time and time again. We can learn a lot about how the healthy brain works from the description people with epilepsy give of their seizures or from observing epileptic seizures.

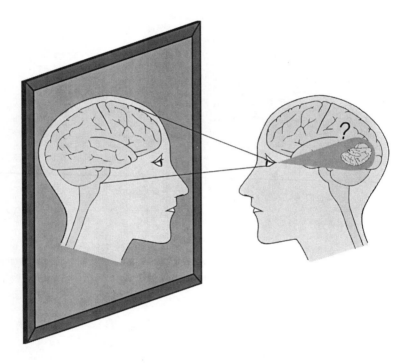

However, we still have much to learn about the workings of the brain. It is fascinating to consider that in this research, one brain examines how another one works. An organ studies itself.

1.5 HOW THE BRAIN WORKS

THE BRAIN RECEIVES SIGNALS FROM THE BODY AND THE OUTSIDE WORLD AND REACTS TO THEM

The eyes translate light into electrical signals. These electrical signals are sent to the brain through the nerves. The brain's reaction mainly goes out to the muscles. For example, the head may turn toward the source of the light.

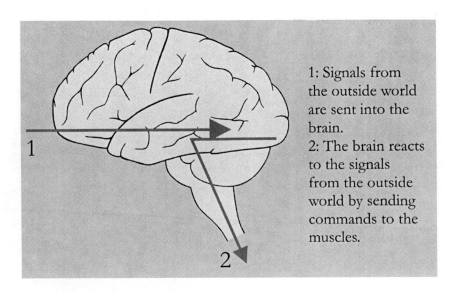

1: Signals from the outside world are sent into the brain.
2: The brain reacts to the signals from the outside world by sending commands to the muscles.

The electrical impulses from the eyes tell the brain where in the outside world light and colors are. The brain uses this information to produce a picture of the real world, which is similar to a photograph.

It is quite well known how the eyes or ears translate light or sounds into electrical signals, and how these signals travel to the brain. The brain translates millions of electrical impulses back into a picture of the outside world.

> During a seizure, the normal electrical activity of the brain is replaced by epileptic activity.

THE BRAIN CONSISTS OF 20,000,000,000 NERVE CELLS

Many of these nerve cells are found close to the surface of the brain, within an outer layer called "cortex" (meaning "bark of a tree"). These nerve cells can be seen through a microscope.

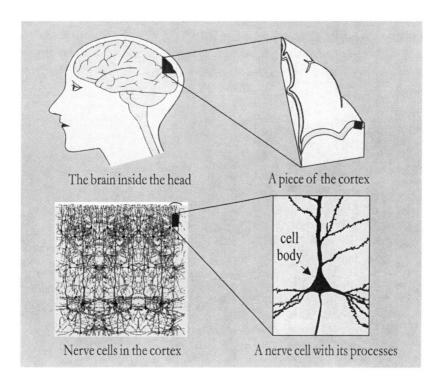

The brain inside the head   A piece of the cortex

cell body

Nerve cells in the cortex   A nerve cell with its processes

The top left part of the picture shows the position of the brain inside the head. The area marked is shown on the right. An enlarged slice (as it is seen through a microscope) is on the bottom left. The area marked is enlarged further on the bottom right. This panel shows a nerve cell with its body and "processes" (fibers). The fibers come out of the cell body. They pick up electrical impulses from other nerve cells and pass them on.

THE SENSORY ORGANS TRANSLATE LIGHT, SOUND, TOUCH, OR HEAT INTO ELECTRICAL ACTIVITY

Nerve cells in sensory organs (like the eyes, ears, and the skin) have fibers with specialized endings. Such endings pick up signals from the outside world and translate them into small amounts of electrical activity. Nerve endings in the ears can pick up sound, while different endings in the eye or skin turn light or touch into electrical activity. The picture shows a nerve ending in the skin. The ending turns pressure applied to the skin into a small amount of electrical activity, which can be measured as a voltage.

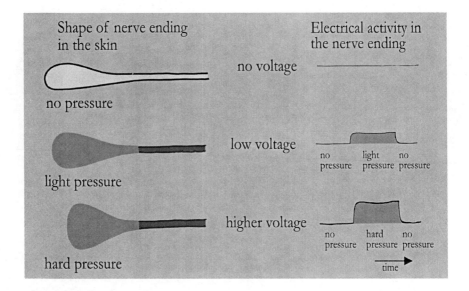

Under light pressure, the skin and the nerve endings in the skin are pulled slightly out of shape. The greater the pressure, the more the nerve endings are pulled. Changing the shape of the ending causes electrical activity, which appears in the nerve fiber. If the pressure on the skin increases, so does the electrical activity. The voltage produced by this electrical tension is shown on the right side of the picture. There are other nerve endings in the skin that react to warmth, and others again that produce electrical activity when the skin is injured.

ELECTRICAL ACTIVITY IS TRANSFORMED INTO ELECTRICAL IMPULSES

Before the amount of electrical activity in the nerve endings can be passed on to the brain, it has to be translated into impulses. Lower voltages are turned into fewer impulses than higher voltages. The picture shows how smaller and larger amounts of electrical activity are translated into impulses. These impulses are called "action potentials."

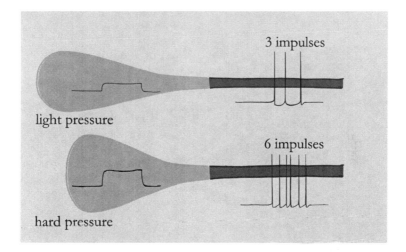

The amount of tension in the nerve endings has to be translated into action potentials because only electrical impulses can travel along the nerve fibers to the brain. Impulses travel very quickly along nerves. When they arrive in the brain, they are translated back into electrical activity.

The electrical activity in the nerve endings can be reduced by cooling. This is why applying ice can help to stop pain from a twisted ankle. Nerves can also be stopped from carrying electrical impulses into the brain. An injection at the dentist, for instance, stops you from feeling pain because the pain impulses cannot reach the brain.

NEIGHBORING NERVE ENDINGS IN THE SKIN ARE CONNECTED TO NEIGHBORING NERVE CELLS IN THE BRAIN

Electrical impulses from two nerve endings next to each other in the skin travel next to each other in a nerve and reach areas close to each other in the outer layers of the brain. This is the "localization principle of information processing." The picture shows how this principle works. On the left is an area of skin with nerve endings seen from inside the body.

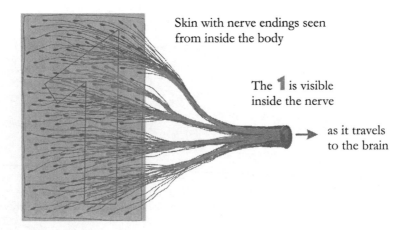

Skin with nerve endings seen from inside the body

The **1** is visible inside the nerve

as it travels to the brain

The number 1 is pressed lightly onto the skin. The number is made from wood and is about 10 cm long. The picture shows the area where the skin is pulled out of its usual shape by the wooden number 1. The nerve endings build up electrical activity because of the pressure in this area. The electrical activity is translated into electrical impulses that travel along the nerve fibers to the brain. A nerve, consisting of many fibers, has been cut through on the right side of the picture. If the fibers carrying electrical impulses inside this nerve were to light up, an image of the number 1 would appear within the nerve (shown in the picture). The nerve fibers would light up as long as the wooden number 1 was pressed onto the skin.

A PICTURE OF THE OUTSIDE WORLD IS PUT TOGETHER IN THE OUTER LAYERS OF THE BRAIN

Initially, the outside world (light, sound, heat, etc.) is pictured in the sensory organs. The organs produce electrical activity and send it to the brain. In the brain, this electrical activity makes up a picture of the outside world.

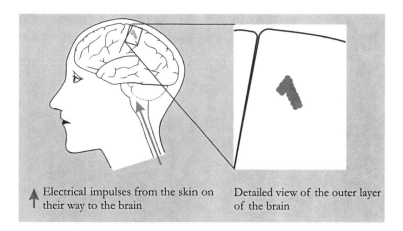

Electrical impulses from the skin on their way to the brain

Detailed view of the outer layer of the brain

As an example, the wooden number 1 is pictured in the outer layers of the brain. This is possible because nerve endings from neighboring areas of skin send electrical impulses to neighboring areas of the brain. If someone loses a leg, the area of the brain that dealt with sensations from the leg is still okay. This means that some people can still feel pain in the leg although the leg actually no longer exists. In contrast, when the surface of the brain linked to the leg is gone, people may feel that their leg does not belong to them, although there is nothing wrong with the leg itself. If the vision center of the brain is damaged, people lose their vision although their eyes work normally.

Each point on the surface of the body is connected to particular points in the outer layers of the brain.

PICKING UP, STORING, AND RETRIEVING MEMORIES

The nerve cells of the brain also deal with learning and memory. It is not entirely clear how they do this. There is, however, evidence that there are two different types of memory stores, "working" (or "short-term" memory) and "long-term" memory. The working memory will only hold on to new facts for a few seconds. Everything we experience right now is contained in the working memory. Important new facts and experiences are moved to the long-term memory. Having the same experience several times makes it more likely that it will be stored in the long-term memory.

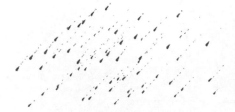 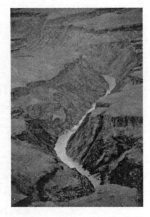

Each drop of rain leaves a small trace. Many rain drops together shape the "long-term memory" of the earth.

Information held in the working memory center is moved to long-term memory stores by the hippocampus. It is more difficult to move information if the hippocampus is damaged in both halves of the brain. Such a problem with storing new memories does not change the way people experience life as it happens. They only find it harder to remember things after 5 minutes or 2 days. For instance, people who fall over and hurt themselves would normally commit the fall to their long-term memory, so that they would be able to remember it later. Someone with damage to the left and right hippocampus would have just as much pain after the fall but may not remember the fall or the pain later.

CONSCIOUSNESS

Consciousness is the clarity with which we are aware of the world around us. This clarity may be reduced or absent altogether. It is related to the perception of the world by the brain, not by the eyes. People can be unconscious while their eyes are open and they appear to be awake.

There are different types of seizures in which consciousness is reduced or lost completely. For instance, consciousness is always reduced or absent in complex partial seizures. Simple actions like laughing or fiddling with clothes may still be carried out during such a seizure, but they would not be remembered later. The pictures show how consciousness may be clouded or lost completely.

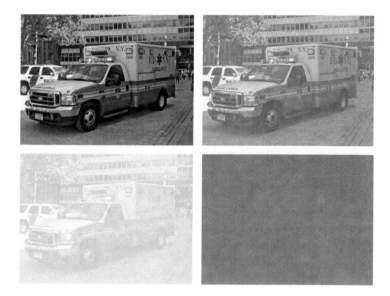

With permission from Thomas Link

There are still many questions about how the brain produces consciousness or learning and memory. About 40 years ago, it was noted that consciousness could be split into a consciousness of the right and left halves of the brain if the fibers connecting the two hemispheres were cut. The two halves of the brain are slightly different. In most people, for instance, only the left half of the brain can produce speech, but both halves are able to read.

NORMALLY, THE NERVE CELLS IN THE BRAIN APPEAR TO FIRE CHAOTICALLY

Activity of nerve cells in the outer layers of the brain varies under normal conditions. Each nerve cell is more or less active, depending on the number of electrical impulses it has received from the sensory organs or on what someone is doing at the time. In the picture, electrical activity is shown as spots. The whole surface of the brain lights up. Taking a closer look, the spots are not spread evenly over the surface of the brain.

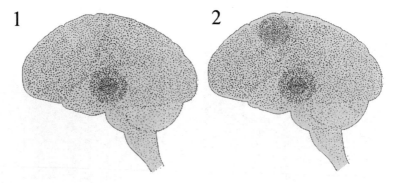

Dots showing electrical activity

The dots are stronger in active areas of the brain. The person whose brain is shown in picture 1 is listening to music. The person whose brain is shown in picture 2 is dancing to the music, so the hearing and movement areas of the brain are particularly active.

Movements are also caused by electrical activity in nerve cells, which send electrical impulses ("action potentials") to the muscles. The more action potentials that reach the muscle, the stronger the movement.

> Muscles close to each other are controlled by neighboring areas in the brain.

1.6 WHAT HAPPENS IN THE BRAIN DURING AN EPILEPTIC SEIZURE?

NERVE CELLS NORMALLY PRODUCE ELECTRICAL IMPULSES FROM TIME TO TIME

The picture shows two series of action potentials (impulses), which come from two neighboring nerve cells in the brain. Each upright line is one action potential.

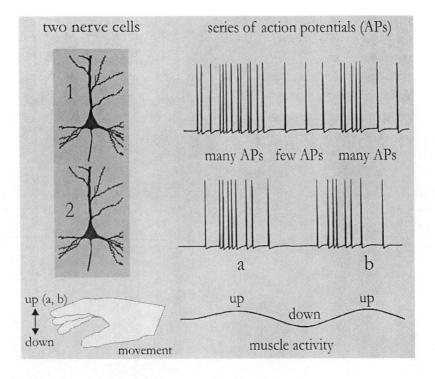

The picture shows the action potentials produced by a nerve cell in the movement area of the brain. The action potentials from this cell travel to a muscle. Each action potential makes the muscle twitch slightly. Many small twitches merge into a movement. If more action potentials reach the muscle, it will tense up more strongly. Two series of action potentials traveling to the muscles of a finger, for instance, will cause the movements marked "a" and "b" in the picture.

DURING A SEIZURE, NORMAL ELECTRICAL IMPULSES ARE REPLACED BY EPILEPTIC ACTIVITY

This picture shows two epileptic potentials of nerve cell 1 and two potentials of nerve cell 2, marked in a darker shade. The epileptic potentials in the two cells appear at the same time.

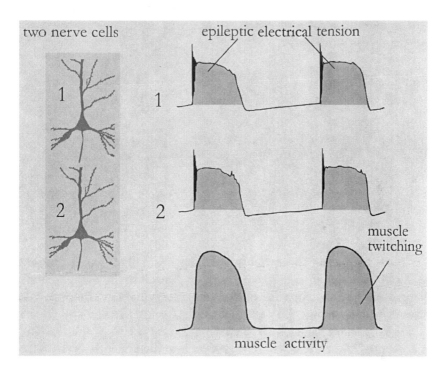

If epileptic activity occurs in nerve cells linked to muscles, electrical impulses are carried from the cells to the muscles. They make the muscle tense up (in a tonic seizure) or jerk (in a clonic seizure). Nerve cells may send out many electrical impulses to the muscles during an epileptic seizure, so that the muscle contraction can be very strong. Epileptic activity can affect many cells at the same time, so that most muscles of the body may tense up and relax in turn. People cannot control the movements of their muscles during this sort of epileptic seizure.

DURING EPILEPTIC ACTIVITY, ALL AFFECTED NERVE CELLS ARE MARCHING IN STEP

The normal activity of nerve cells is like "chaotic chatter." In contrast, during epileptic activity, all affected nerve cells send out electrical impulses at the same time and are "silent" in between.

As more and more nerve cells march in step, the area of the brain producing epileptic activity increases. In line with this, the seizure involves a greater area of the body.

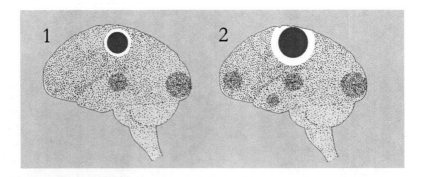

In picture 1, most of the brain is working normally. This is shown by the dots. Although an epileptic seizure has started in the movement area of the brain and the muscles of the arm are twitching, the person can see and hear normally. The area of the brain involved in the epileptic activity is marked in black. It is surrounded by a rim of white. This is an area in which nerve cells are trying to stop the epileptic activity from spilling over to the rest of the brain.

In picture 2, the area of the brain affected by the epileptic activity has grown. The twitching does not only affect the arm now, but also the shoulder. Over the next few seconds, the epileptic activity can shrink back. However, it can also spread further.

Epileptic activity interrupts the normal working of the brain.

PARTS OF THE BRAIN NOT AFFECTED BY EPILEPTIC ACTIVITY WORK NORMALLY DURING A SEIZURE

It is possible that an epileptic seizure can cause someone to have muscle twitches or see flashes of light, but they may have no trouble with hearing or speaking. However, epileptic activity involving only one part of the brain (as in a focal seizure) can spread to involve the whole brain, leading to "secondary generalization."

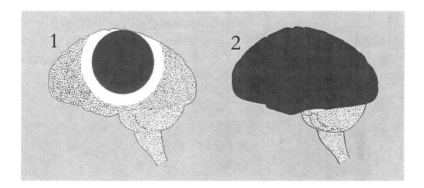

Picture 1 shows epileptic activity affecting a large part of the brain. It is marked in black. Picture 2 shows epileptic activity in both halves of the brain. If epileptic activity involves the whole brain, then perception, thinking, and consciousness are interrupted. The person having the seizure will have no memory of it and will be unable to react to speech or touch during the seizure.

Most seizures stop by themselves. In some cases, they do not stop and status epilepticus develops. Status epilepticus is a medical emergency. It has to be treated immediately. If a seizure goes on for longer than 5 minutes, an ambulance should be called.

It is not clear why epileptic activity starts and stops.

"HIGHER MENTAL FUNCTIONS" OF THE BRAIN AND EPILEPSY

It is not clear exactly how the brain performs complicated tasks like perception, thinking, attention, and memory, and how these tasks relate to intelligence. Many of these so-called "higher mental functions" of the brain are not performed by specialized, single centers in the brain, but by different brain regions working together in networks.

Brain cells do not work in their normal manner when they produce epileptic activity. If epileptic activity affects the whole outer layer of the brain, then all higher functions are switched off and consciousness is lost. However, in between seizures, when there is no epileptic activity, the brain usually works normally unless there is another problem separate from the seizures that affects brain function. It is therefore not surprising that most people with epilepsy can do all kinds of jobs.

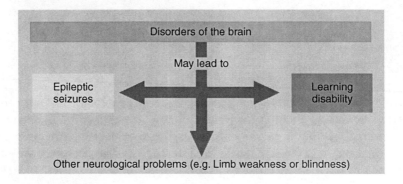

Some people with learning disabilities also have epilepsy, but epilepsy does not cause learning disabilities. Epileptic seizures do not damage brain cells. (One exception to this is status epilepticus with tonic-clonic seizures, which is a life-threatening condition). Sometimes, however, a disorder of the brain leads to both epilepsy and learning disability.

MEMORY AND EPILEPSY

Some people with epilepsy have poor memory. Memory problems are particularly common when epileptic seizures are caused by damage to the temporal lobes. The temporal lobes contain the hippocampus. The hippocampus is a part of the brain that is particularly important for memory functions. It lies close to the center of the skull and can be damaged during complicated febrile seizures in childhood or status epilepticus in adults. The hippocampus acts like a temporary store for information waiting to be secured as more permanent memories, or for memories retrieved from permanent stores and brought to a person's attention. It can be compared to a warehouse that holds raw materials going into a factory and finished goods waiting to be shipped out.

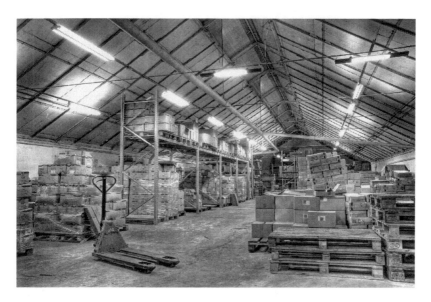

With permission from Robert Smolenski (rsmolens@gmail.com)

A damaged hippocampus often causes temporal lobe epilepsy. Seizures can stop when the hippocampus is removed. Operations on the hippocampus sometimes make memory problems worse. This cannot always be predicted before epilepsy surgery is undertaken.

Memory problems can also be caused by the drugs used to treat seizures. Phenobarbital and primidone in particular are known to affect memory.

THE CAUSE OF EPILEPSY CANNOT BE FOUND IN EVERYONE

At present, it is only possible to identify the cause of epileptic seizures in 4 or 5 out of every 10 people with epilepsy. For instance, a scar from a brain injury can cause epileptic seizures. If this is the case, epileptic activity develops around the scar. We do not know how a scar can change the way nerve cells work so that they begin to cause epileptic seizures. We also do not know why seizures from the scar only happen from time to time. Similar events in nature can help us to understand these things better.

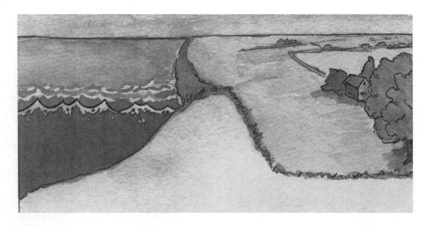

In this picture, living with epilepsy is compared to living close to the sea. Water can spill over the dam if the sea level rises, the waves become bigger, or the dam becomes smaller. In this picture, the tendency to have epileptic seizures is represented by the level of the sea. If the waves are small, no water will spill onto the land (there will be no seizures) even if the sea level is high (there is a strong tendency to have an epileptic seizure). If the size of the waves increases, water may spill over the dam (a seizure may happen). Using this analogy, antiepileptic drugs can stop seizures by calming the waves or by building up the size of the dam.

2

RECOGNIZING EPILEPSY

2.1 FIRST TESTS

IS IT EPILEPSY AT ALL?

If someone has their first blackout or "episode," they may see a doctor for advice. The doctor will first try to work out whether the problem is likely to have come from the brain and could be a form of epilepsy, or whether the symptoms were caused by a totally different problem. There will be many questions that will help in this first assessment.

What happens during the episode?

If the episode struck suddenly and lasted no longer than a few minutes, it may have been a seizure. The seizure may have been caused by epilepsy or another problem. To find out the cause, a clear description of the episode is needed. What does the person who had it remember? Did anyone else see it happen? What did they notice? It is particularly important to find out what happened from witnesses, if the episode actually caused a blackout. Were there any movements after consciousness was lost? Was the body stiff or floppy? If it was floppy during a blackout, the attack may not have been caused by epilepsy.

Are there repeated episodes?

There are epileptic seizures that happen only once in a lifetime or very rarely. An example is "febrile seizures." Febrile seizures are seizures that affect some young children when they have a high temperature. Such seizures would not normally be treated with taking antiepileptic drugs on a daily basis. If the triggers for provoked seizures are avoided, they may not happen at all. A diagnosis of epilepsy would only be made if seizures happened repeatedly and without provocation.

Have attacks happened before?

Epileptic seizures are usually very similar in one person. If the appearance of episodes changes a lot, it is less likely that they are caused by epilepsy. Sometimes they are caused by stress or difficulties with handling thoughts, memories, or feelings and not by epileptic discharges in the brain. Such episodes are called "non-epileptic," "psychogenic," or "functional" seizures. Some types of attack are typical for a certain age; absence seizures for example are most likely to occur in childhood.

Does the episode spread from one part of the body to another?

The answer to this question can help classify epileptic seizures into focal or "primary generalized" seizures. A primary generalized seizure occurs when electrical discharges begin in both halves of the brain at the same time. In a "secondary generalized seizure," the seizure starts in one half of the body (and one half of the brain) but then spreads to the other.

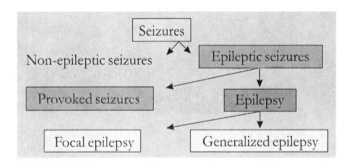

At the first visit, the doctor gets some idea of the nature of the episodes. The diagram shows which decisions have to be made. Was it a seizure? Was it caused by epilepsy? Was the seizure provoked? What was the seizure type?

A GOOD DESCRIPTION OF THE SEIZURES IS VERY IMPORTANT

What happened the day before the seizure? What happened in the minutes leading up to it? Was there lack of sleep, stress, or some other problem? What happened during the seizure? What did the movements look like? Were the eyes open or closed? Every detail matters. For instance, did the seizure start with little twitches in the fingers of one hand spreading up the hand, arm, and shoulder, or was there a sudden blackout without warning, followed by a fall and a convulsion? If seizures happen frequently, it is sometimes possible for friends or family members to make a video recording or to take photographs of the seizure. This can be very helpful.

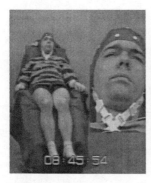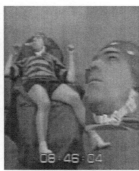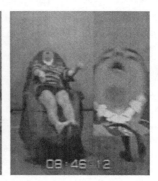

The picture shows single frames from a video recording, which was made in a hospital. The first picture shows a man shortly before a seizure. He is relaxing in a chair. The second picture shows the beginning of a seizure. This man feels as if his head and eyes are pulled over to the right side. At this point, he loses consciousness. The third picture shows that the seizure has turned into a secondary generalized tonic-clonic seizure. The time code on the video frames demonstrates that the third picture was recorded 18 seconds after the first.

SEIZURES CANNOT BE STOPPED BY AN OBSERVER

An epileptic seizure cannot be stopped by people who are present at the time. Seizures will run their course and stop after some seconds or minutes. Of course, witnesses to a seizure should make sure that the person having it is safe. Things that could be dangerous, a burning candle or a piece of furniture for instance, should be moved out of the way. However, it does not help the person with epilepsy if other people panic during a seizure. Epileptic seizures can look frightening, but it is important that people try to stay calm. If possible, observers should look at their watch and time the seizure.

Absence seizure		
no warning	short blackout without fall	quick recovery

Complex partial seizure		
Warning, aura	not answering, fiddling, licking lips	gradual recovery

Tonic-clonic seizure		
no warning, no aura	convulsion of the whole body	exhaustion, tiredness

How people feel after a seizure depends on the seizure type. After a tonic-clonic seizure, people are very achy and tired. After a complex partial seizure, people can be confused, may not recognize their family or friends, or know where they are. This kind of confusion may not be obvious until they are spoken to. It is therefore best not to leave someone on their own after such a seizure. On the other hand, absence seizures stop as suddenly as they start. After an absence seizure, people immediately know where they are, and what they were doing. A description of what happened shortly after a seizure can help to classify it.

OBSERVATION AND DESCRIPTION ALLOW A SEIZURE TO BE CLASSIFIED

The classification of seizures used at present is based on ideas developed over the past few hundred years. The diagram shows the classification of the International League Against Epilepsy (ILAE). The ILAE is an organization of scientists and clinicians with a special interest in epilepsy. It has branches in many countries.

Partial seizures	Generalized seizures
Focal sensory seizures – with elementary symptoms – with experiential symptoms	Absence seizures
	Myoclonic seizures
Focal motor seizures – with clonic signs – with tonic signs – with automatisms	Tonic seizures
	Clonic seizures
	Tonic-clonic seizures
Secondary generalized seizures	Atonic seizures

The diagram shows the main headings of the current classification of seizures. Today the word "focal" in the latest version of the classification means the same as the terms "partial" or "localization-related." The correct classification of these seizures helps people with epilepsy because it makes it easier to choose a suitable antiepileptic drug. It is also important for specialists because it helps them to understand each other better when they discuss certain types of epilepsy.

A NEUROLOGICAL EXAMINATION SHOWS WHETHER THERE ARE OTHER PROBLEMS WITH THE BRAIN

During a neurological examination, the many functions of the brain (and the rest of the nervous system) are tested with very simple means. Just comparing the muscles and skin of the right half of the body with the left can sometimes give a clue to a problem with the brain. Movements may also look different on the two sides. After a stroke, for instance, people may drag one leg (strokes are not caused by epilepsy, but sometimes a scar from a stroke can cause epileptic seizures). When the reflexes are tested, the tendons are stretched a little by the tap of a rubber hammer. Again, the reflexes on the right are compared to those on the left.

Such simple tests paint a picture of the brain in the doctor's mind. Often the examination is completely normal in people with epilepsy.

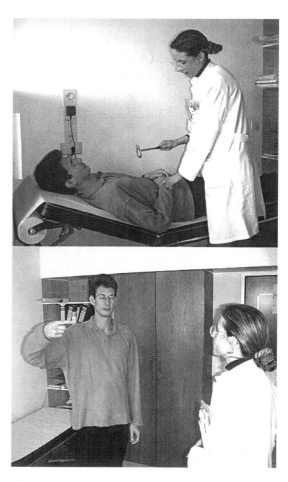

The top picture shows an examination of the reflexes. The picture at the bottom shows the finger-nose test. In this test, the patient is asked to touch the tip of his nose with his index finger, with his eyes open at first, then with his eyes closed. In some conditions, patients struggle with this test.

INITIAL BLOOD TESTS

Blood flows through all parts of the body. When it flows through a part of the body that is not working well, the composition of the blood can change. Sometimes these changes can be detected and provide a clue to the underlying disease. Several diseases, including tumors, infection, or problems with the body's metabolism, can cause epileptic seizures. Blood tests can sometimes help to find out about such conditions.

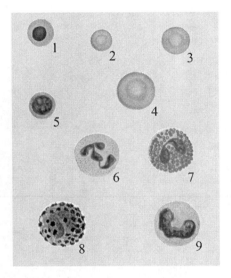

This is a picture of blood cells. Cell number 1 is not normally seen in the blood. The cell numbers 2–4 are red blood cells. These are the commonest cells in the blood. The cell numbers 5–9 are white blood cells that have been stained so that one cell type can be distinguished from another.

The diets of some people do not contain enough vitamin B. People who regularly drink too much alcohol, for instance, can suffer from a lack of vitamin B. This causes the cells in the blood to change. A blood film may show red blood cells with a nucleus inside them (cell number 1), red cells that are larger than usual (cell number 4), and fewer white cells than there should be (5–9). A lack of vitamin B can also cause seizures. If vitamins are taken, the seizures can improve, and the blood cells look normal again.

PROBLEMS WITH THE BODY'S METABOLISM CAN CAUSE EPILEPTIC SEIZURES

The body is made up of many different substances, which are broken down and put together again. This constant activity (the body's metabolism) can be compared to a system of assembly lines on which more complicated substances are made out of more basic ones (picture on the left). When one particular assembly line is jammed (picture on the right), two problems arise. First, there is a lack of the more complicated substance (1). Second, the basic substances are not used up, so that they pile up (2) in the body's tissues. If the unused material is stored in the brain, it can damage the nerve cells and cause epileptic seizures. Blood and urine tests can help to recognize such storage diseases.

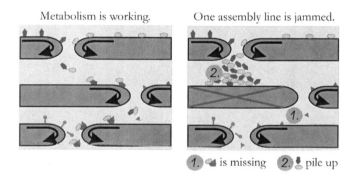

Metabolism is working.   One assembly line is jammed.

1. ◀ is missing   2. ⦂ pile up

Phenylketonuria is an example of a problem with the body's metabolism. The illness often causes epileptic seizures in the first few years of life. It affects the development of the brain. If children are put on a special diet early on, seizures can be prevented and the brain can develop more normally.

Blood tests can show whether the body's organs or metabolism are working well.

NOT ALL SEIZURES ARE EPILEPTIC

A person faints (also called syncope) when there is a problem with the supply of blood and oxygen to the brain. A lack of oxygen to the brain can cause collapses and blackouts that may look similar to epileptic seizures. However, people often feel light-headed and queasy for several minutes before fainting, whereas there is usually only a very short warning (if any) before an epileptic seizure. People also come around much more quickly after a faint than a seizure. Sometimes a collapse and blackout can also be caused by stress or a problem with handling painful memories, thoughts, or emotions. Such attacks may look quite similar to epilepsy and be wrongly treated with antiepileptic drugs for many years.

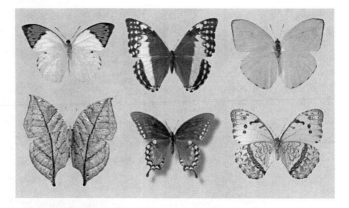

The picture shows an example of a mix up that may happen in nature. Leaves are rarely mistaken for butterflies. However, you have to take a close look not to confuse the butterfly in the bottom left-hand corner with two leaves.

However, in most cases it is not difficult to diagnose epilepsy.

2.2 EEG

THE EEG CAN HELP IN THE DIAGNOSIS OF EPILEPSY

The EEG (electroencephalogram) picks up electrical activity from the surface of the brain through small metal plates (electrodes), which are attached to the scalp. The EEG can be recorded on paper with a printer, or it may be stored on a computer and studied on a computer screen. A full EEG examination takes about 1 hour. It does not hurt and is without any risk. At first, the electrodes have to be positioned on the skin using rubber straps or a special glue. It is important that people having an EEG are calm and relaxed because muscle tension can hide electrical activity from the brain.

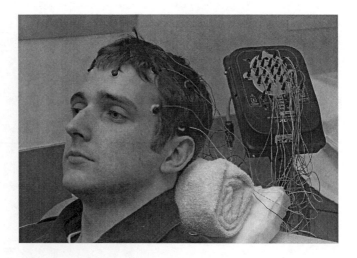

What the EEG does not show

The EEG was invented by Hans Berger in 1932. He hoped that it would allow him to record people's thoughts. However, thoughts, feelings, or intelligence cannot be measured with the EEG. When the EEG is recorded, it is merely possible to see *whether* a person might be thinking, but not *what* they are thinking about.

Each electrode is wired to one of the ink pens of the EEG machine or one of the EEG lines on a computer screen. This line shows the electrical activity underneath the particular electrode on the scalp. If the electrical activity underneath the electrode changes, it makes the line on the printer or the computer screen move, so that it ends up showing a wavy line for each of the electrodes. During an epileptic seizure, the EEG may show typical epileptic activity, depending on the location of the seizure in the brain.

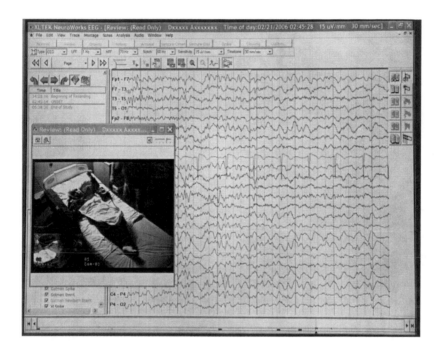

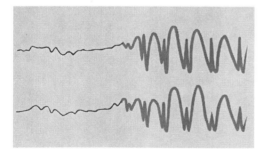

The EEG is mainly used to support the diagnosis of epilepsy or to see whether changes in the EEG have occurred over time.

This picture shows electrical activity from the brain recorded from two electrodes. The right side of the recording (bold part) shows electrical activity typical of a seizure.

THE ELECTRICAL SIGNALS OF MANY NERVE CELLS TOGETHER MAKE UP THE WAVES OF THE EEG

The waves of the EEG show a typical pattern when the eyes are open and a different pattern when the eyes are closed. The shapes of the waves are shown in the picture.

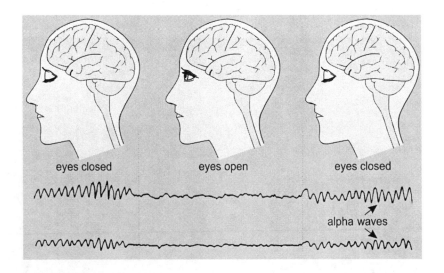

The waves, which are normally seen when someone is fully relaxed with their eyes closed, are called alpha waves. They disappear when the eyes are opened or the person thinks about something. In every EEG examination, the waves are checked with the eyes open and closed.

Example

Mr. A. had been having headaches for 1 week. He was also quite irritable and found it hard to concentrate. Then, one morning, his wife found it difficult to wake him up. He hardly responded when she talked to him or prodded him. When Mr. A. arrived at the hospital in this state, an EEG showed widespread slow activity. Mr. A. was diagnosed with encephalitis. After he had been given treatment for several days, he was alert again and reacted normally when people spoke to him. The EEG then showed normal alpha waves.

FOCAL EPILEPSY MAY ONLY PRODUCE ABNORMAL SIGNALS IN A SINGLE EEG ELECTRODE

In the picture, electrode number (1) "looks" at a part of the brain surface that deals with sensation in the face. A person with epileptic activity in this area may feel a tingling sensation or an unusual pressure in one part of his or her face. Isolated epileptic signals may also be picked up in the EEG in this area when the person is not aware of any abnormal sensations in his/her face. These are also called "interictal" (between seizures) "epileptiform" abnormalities.

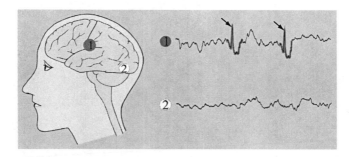

Tall, sharp potentials (also called spikes) are a typical EEG signal of focal seizures. If the epileptic area (or focus) in the brain was larger, the spikes seen under electrode number (1) would also be seen in electrode (2). Some people have several separate areas where the brain shows epileptic activity. If there were two separate epileptic areas rather than one large area, spikes would appear in electrode (1) and (2) at different times.

Example

An 18-year-old man had his first seizure at the age of 4. After this, he had no seizures for 10 years, then seizures started again. An EEG recorded while he was sleeping showed tall and pointed signals under the area marked by a dark spot in the picture. Occasionally, he has tonic-clonic seizures, during which epileptic activity spreads to the rest of the brain from this area. So far, drugs have failed to stop his seizures.

Example

Mrs. S. had meningitis when she was 10 years old. She was very ill with fever, headache, and vomiting. Shortly after these symptoms stopped, she developed several different types of epileptic seizures. Mrs S. takes a combination of antiepileptic drugs, which have stopped her from having tonic-clonic seizures. She had no seizures while undergoing an EEG examination.

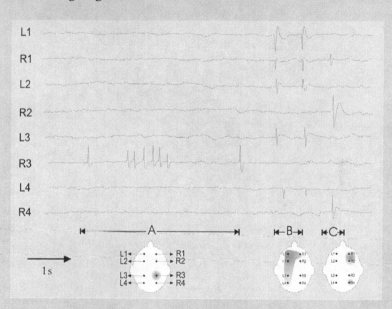

The EEG was recorded from four electrodes on the left side of the head (L1–L4) and four electrodes on the right side of the head (R1–R4). The pictures at the bottom of the diagram show Mrs. S.'s head from above. They indicate where the electrodes were placed. These pictures (A, B, and C) also indicate where epileptic activity was picked up during the different times of the recording. During period A, epileptic changes are only seen in electrode R3. During period B, spikes are seen in a larger area covered by electrodes L1–L4 and R1. During period C, changes are seen in R1, R2, and R4. The findings suggest that Mrs. S.'s seizures start in different parts of the brain. She has "multifocal" epilepsy.

GENERALIZED EPILEPSY PRODUCES ABNORMAL SIGNALS IN BOTH HALVES OF THE BRAIN

In this picture, epileptic activity is recorded from electrodes over all the brain areas. While this activity is recorded, consciousness is lost. The EEG shows a brief absence seizure. During this type of epileptic seizure, people seem to "freeze" for a few seconds.

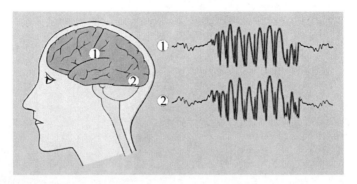

The EEG can show whether epileptic activity occurs in all electrodes from the very beginning of a seizure (as in primary generalized seizures) or whether it starts in one electrode and then spreads to others (as in partial seizures with secondary generalization). This is very important, because the two types of epilepsy are treated differently.

Example

A 5-year-old girl developed short blackouts (absence seizures) during which she was unconscious but did not fall or move. During such attacks, the EEG showed the pattern of spikes and waves marked bold in the picture. Her seizures stopped when she started to take an antiepileptic drug. When there had been no seizures for several years, she decided to try to reduce the medication with her doctor's help.

For some years, twelve-year-old Paul has had brief moments during which he stares into space. He seems to come around rapidly when he is spoken to, so his family, friends, and teachers thought that he was just absentminded. Eventually, Paul had a tonic-clonic seizure and underwent an EEG. This showed that his moments of absentmindedness were epileptic absence seizures.

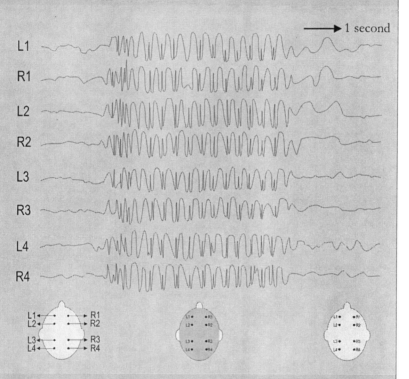

The EEG was recorded with eight electrodes (L1 to L4 and R1 to R4). The picture at the bottom of the diagram shows where the electrodes were attached to the head. The EEG suddenly became abnormal in all electrodes. Paul did not answer when the technician tried to talk to him. The abnormal signals disappeared again after 6 seconds. Paul could not remember that the technician had tried to speak to him.

MANY PEOPLE WITH EPILEPSY HAVE A NORMAL EEG BETWEEN SEIZURES

The EEG describes what happens in the outer layer of the brain during the EEG recording. When there is no epileptic activity during the recording, the EEG may be normal. When there is epileptic activity, the EEG shows typical EEG waves such as "spikes" and "sharp waves," which show that a person is at higher risk of having epileptic seizures. A normal EEG docs not exclude epilepsy. On the other hand, some people who have abnormal brain waves do not have seizures.

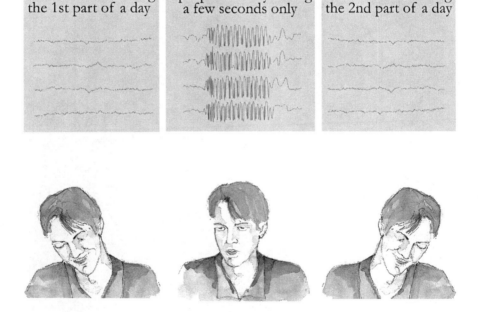

Normal EEG during the 1st part of a day

Epileptic activity lasting a few seconds only

Normal EEG during the 2nd part of a day

In some people with epilepsy, abnormal brain waves can be "provoked." During an EEG recording, flashing lights or several minutes of deep breathing (hyperventilation) can trigger such brain waves. Recording such EEG changes can be helpful because it can confirm the diagnosis and may identify the type of seizure disorder. The diagnosis of epilepsy does not only depend on the results of the EEG but also on the description of the episode(s).

THE EEG MAY NEED TO BE REPEATED

There are many reasons for repeating an EEG on a different day:

- The first EEG only included wakefulness and was normal.
- The chance of picking up diagnostic changes in the EEG is higher during a sleep EEG recording.
- Using a small recorder, which is worn on a waist belt, the EEG can be recorded over a period of one or more days. An account of daily activities and symptoms helps in the interpretation of EEG changes.
- An EEG recording may help in understanding why seizures have changed or become more frequent.
- An EEG linked to a video camera can show movements of the patient and brain wave patterns simultaneously. Both signals are stored on a computer and analyzed together. When surgery is being considered to stop epileptic seizures, special electrodes may be used that are stuck under the skin using a small needle ("sphenoidal electrodes"). The use of such electrodes can be unpleasant. In all other cases, EEG recordings are painless and not harmful.

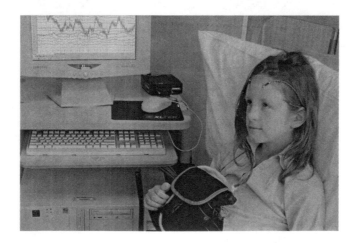

SPECIAL EEG RECORDINGS MAY BE NECESSARY WHEN EPILEPSY SURGERY IS BEING CONSIDERED

The brain's electrical activity fluctuates from second to second, but routine EEGs provide only a 20- to 40-minute sample of brain wave activity. If epileptic activity occurs only once every 3 or 4 hours, or if it appears only after an hour of sleep, for instance, a routine EEG may be normal. Then the doctor may want to see a longer recording that includes periods of wakefulness and sleep. This kind of recording is called an ambulatory EEG. "Ambulatory" means that people may walk around during the recording.

An ambulatory EEG may be performed to confirm the diagnosis of epilepsy if seizures have continued despite seizure medicines. It would usually be available at a specialized epilepsy center.

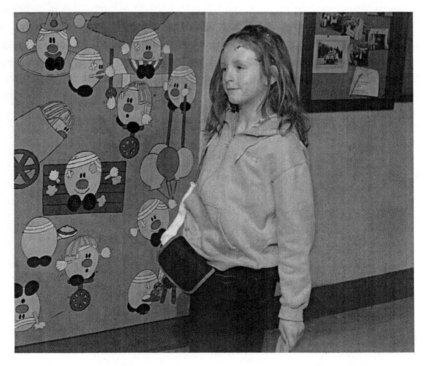

With an ambulatory EEG, people can go about their normal routine.

This kind of recording is made using a special recorder that is slightly larger than a portable cassette player. It can be attached to a waist belt, with the wires running under the clothes to the head. Then people can go about their normal routine for up to 24 hours or longer. The electrodes can be covered with a hat.

Because the electrodes must stay on the head longer than for a regular EEG, the technologist will probably use a special glue to keep them in place. The glue can be dissolved with a special solution at the end of the test.

Most recorders have an "event" button to press if there are any symptoms for which people are being tested, such as feeling "spaced out" or confused. The button can also be pressed by someone who witnesses a possible seizure. Some home EEG systems can even record video.

The recording of epileptic seizures with an EEG machine is particularly important if seizures don't stop with medication and if epilepsy surgery is being considered. Deciding whether or not a person is likely to benefit from epilepsy surgery is a complicated and often quite lengthy process. It involves not only EEG testing but also a range of other tests. All this information has to be considered together with a detailed history of the epilepsy by a specialized epilepsy surgery team before a final decision about surgery can be made.

EEG AND VIDEO CAN BE RECORDED SIMULTANEOUSLY

In video-EEG, video and EEG can be recorded at the same time. The patient is videotaped at the same time as the EEG is recorded. Video pictures and EEG images can be analyzed together on one computer screen. In this way, it can be seen how the behavior during seizures is related to the electrical activity in the brain. The EEG electrodes are attached to the head using a special glue for this test. People undergoing video-EEG monitoring are encouraged to stay in front of the video camera. This can be quite tedious, because the monitoring may continue for 1 or 2 weeks. Video-EEG is most helpful in determining whether seizures are caused by epileptic discharges or other processes, identifying the type of seizures, and pinpointing the region of the brain where seizures begin. This is particularly important when epilepsy surgery is being considered.

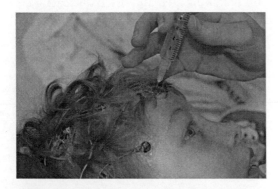

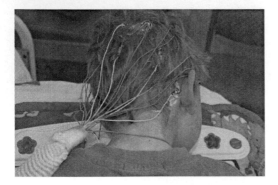

Video-EEG is usually performed in a hospital setting, so that the person can be observed around the clock. The purpose of the monitoring is to record seizure activity. Therefore, seizure medicine is often reduced or stopped by physicians in order to provoke seizures. This is associated with a certain risk of seizures, related injuries, and prolonged seizures and so is only done safely in a specialized hospital setting.

The inspection of video-EEG recordings also requires expertise, so that video-EEG recordings cannot be performed in most hospitals.

OTHER MEDICAL DISORDERS CAN CAUSE CHANGES IN THE EEG

The EEG is mostly used to find out more about the type of epilepsy, where seizures are coming from in the brain, or how well antiepileptic drugs are working. But the EEG can also show changes in association with other conditions that affect brain function.

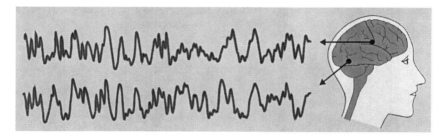

Slow waves of different frequencies with an infection of the brain

Example

A 10-year-old boy was unconscious when he was brought to the hospital. An EEG recording showed irregular slow waves. The EEG changes suggested that the boy had an infection of the brain (encephalitis).

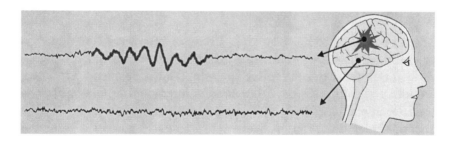

Slow waves near an area of bleeding

Example

Mr. P. developed a sudden and severe headache. The EEG showed slow waves under one electrode. A brain scan showed that a blood vessel had burst in this area of the brain.

THE EEG IS NOT A GOOD TEST TO EXAMINE THE STRUCTURE OF THE BRAIN

The EEG is mostly used to find out more about the type of epilepsy, where seizures are coming from in the brain, or how well antiepileptic drugs are working. The EEG does not produce a very clear picture of the shape or structure of the brain. When it is important to know exactly where seizures start in the brain, information from the EEG (a test of brain function) is combined with information from brain scans (tests of brain structure).

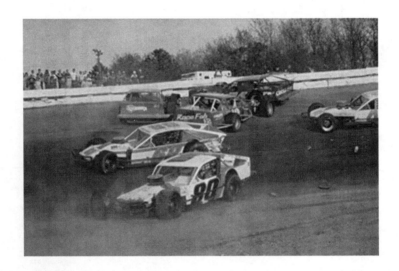

A car can be used to illustrate the difference between a functional and structural problem. Some cars may look broken on the outside but still work (they have a structural but not a functional problem). Other cars look okay but do not work (they have a functional problem, but their structure might look fine). It is particularly important to know about functional and structural problems when epilepsy surgery is being considered. Surgery is more likely to be successful if problems of structure and function affect the same part of the brain.

2.3 TAKING PICTURES OF THE BRAIN

MAGNETIC RESONANCE IMAGING (MRI) SHOWS THE STRUCTURE OF THE BRAIN

"Magnetic resonance imaging" (also known as "magnetic resonance tomography") is usually called MRI. It was developed in the 1970s.

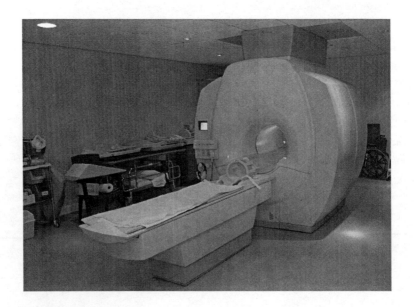

When a brain MRI is performed, the person lies with his/her head inside a strong magnetic field. A scanner then measures the "magnetic resonance" of the head tissues, including the brain. A computer can turn the magnetic signals into a picture of the skull and brain. Each picture shows a slice through the head. The head can be pictured in any direction. This means that abnormalities like scarring of the hippocampus can be seen without opening the skull, even though the hippocampus is on the inside of the temporal lobe of the brain.

Because MRI uses a very strong magnetic field, people who have a pacemaker or other magnetic metals inside their body (like some types of artificial joints or heart valves) cannot be examined with MRI. For other people, MRI is safe and painless.

MRI PRODUCES VERY CLEAR PICTURES OF THE BRAIN

MRI pictures may show small abnormalities that could not be picked up with other methods of imaging the brain. The machine takes 30–60 minutes to record one series of pictures. During this time, the person having the scan has to lie still in a tube that is about 28 inches wide. Some people get anxious because there is little space in the scanner. MRI does not involve X-rays or radiation.

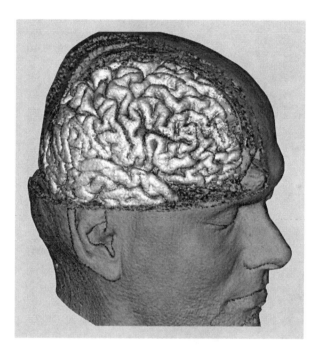

This picture of a man's brain was obtained with an MRI machine and put together by a computer. Since the development of MRI, it has been possible to find changes in the brain in many more people with epilepsy. For example, it is now known that people with complex partial seizures often have scarring of the hippocampus in the temporal lobes.

Not all people with epilepsy need an MRI scan.

MRI PICTURE OF A NORMAL BRAIN

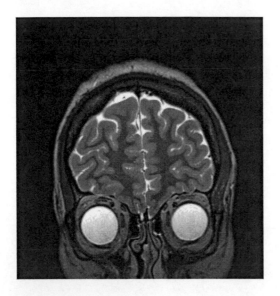

This picture shows the head just behind the forehead. The white circles are the eyes. The brain is shown in gray. The surface of the brain is a little lighter than the center. The skull bone is almost black and can hardly be seen. The light outer rim is the skin.

MRI PICTURE OF A BENIGN TUMOR

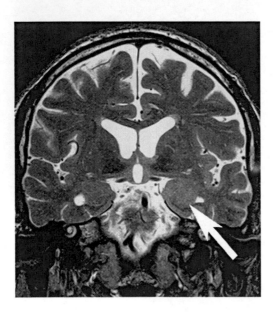

A "benign" (non-cancerous) tumor is marked with an arrow. It is a lighter shade of gray than the brain around it. Sometimes seizures start from the brain tissue around a tumor. They can stop when the tumor is taken out by surgery.

MRI SHOWING SCARRING OF THE BRAIN

The arrow shows a hippocampus that is much smaller than the hippocampus on the other side of the brain. Epileptic seizures often come from this area. Sometimes the hippocampus is damaged many years before seizures start. It can be impossible to identify the cause of a scar like this. This sort of MRI picture is common in people with complex partial seizures.

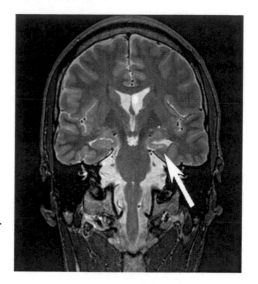

MRI PICTURE SHOWING ABNORMAL DEVELOPMENT OF THE BRAIN

The picture shows a horizontal image of the brain. The arrow marks an area that appears in a lighter shade of gray than the rest of the brain. This area did not develop well when the brain was formed in the womb. It is not made up of normal nerve cells. Such abnormalities are called "cortical malformations," "hamartomas," or "dysplasias." Epileptic seizures can start in the brain tissue around an area of malformation.

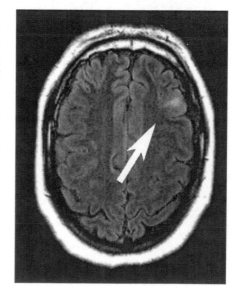

COMPUTED TOMOGRAPHY (CT) CAN ALSO SHOW ABNORMALITIES OF THE SHAPE AND STRUCTURE OF THE BRAIN

Computed tomography, or CT, uses X-rays to take pictures of the skull and brain. X-rays are sent through the head. Special cameras (detectors) pick up to what extent the rays have been weakened by the structures they have passed through in the head. The source of the X-rays and the camera travel around the head. A computer puts all measurements together and produces a picture of the head.

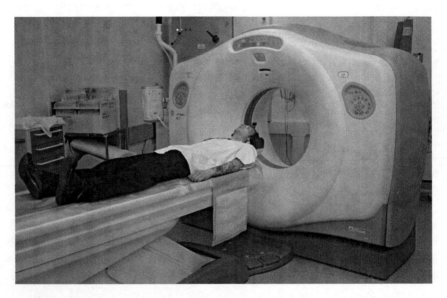

The photo shows a patient having a CT scan. The examination does not hurt and is harmless, although it does involve a small dose of radiation. A CT takes 5–10 minutes. It is important for people to lie still under the CT scanner because otherwise the pictures will not be clear.

CT takes pictures of the brain more quickly than MRI.

CT PICTURE OF A NORMAL BRAIN

This CT picture shows a horizontal image of the brain. The skull bones show up white. The brain appears in shades of gray. The picture of the brain is less clear than that produced by MRI. In the CT, denser structures look brighter than soft ones, whereas in MRI, structures are brighter if they contain more water.

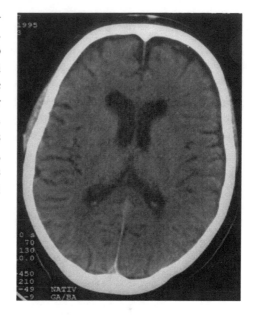

CT PICTURE OF A TUMOR

This picture shows a horizontal image of the brain. The arrow points to a tumor in the frontal lobe. Hypermotor seizures may start from the area of the brain around this tumor. If the tumor is removed by surgery, seizures may stop.

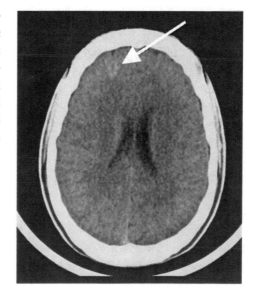

OCCASIONALLY, BLOOD VESSELS HAVE TO BE EXAMINED USING ANGIOGRAPHY

When the MRI or CT pictures suggest that there may be problems with the blood vessels in the brain, these vessels can be examined by angiography. In this test, a dye, which does not let X-rays pass through, is injected into an artery. The blood vessels show up very clearly if an X-ray picture is taken as the dye is injected. Blood vessels can also be imaged using MRI, without the need to inject dye into an artery.

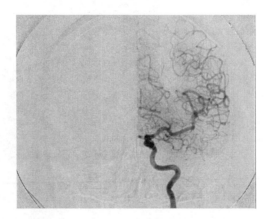

This picture shows a large artery that leads to the right side of the brain.

ANGIOGRAPHY IS SOMETIMES USED BEFORE A BRAIN OPERATION

A brain operation to control seizures is possible if several conditions are met. One condition is that surgery will not damage important functions of the brain. In epilepsy surgery involving the temporal lobes, speech and memory are at particular risk, because they are situated in a region of the brain in which seizures often start. The "Wada test" (named after an epilepsy specialist who developed this test) helps to show whether an operation is likely to affect speech or memory.

The test consists of two steps. At first, the arteries that supply the region to be operated on are evaluated with angiography. A drug is then injected into the artery to put the part of the brain supplied by the artery to sleep. Then, speech and memory are tested. If the person having the test can still understand, speak, and remember with a part of their brain switched off by the drug, then this part can be removed without likely damaging these important functions.

POSITRON EMISSION TOMOGRAPHY (PET) IS SOMETIMES USED IN PEOPLE WITH EPILEPSY

PET pictures show how the brain is working. To take a PET picture, a radioactive substance, for instance a type of sugar, is injected into the blood. The sugar is taken up by the brain. The radiation (or "positrons") sent out by the sugar can be picked up by a special camera outside the body. Areas of the brain that are not working well do not need much sugar, so they show up darker in this test.

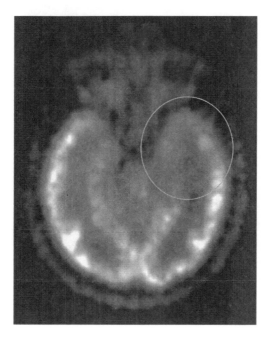

The picture shows a horizontal image of the brain. The brighter the picture, the more sugar has been taken up. The outer layer of the brain, which contains the nerve cells, is particularly busy and needs most sugar. The picture shows a PET scan of a person with right temporal lobe epilepsy. Slightly less sugar was taken up by the area of the brain where seizures come from.

The advantage of PET lies in the fact that it shows not only the structure but also the function of the brain. The disadvantages are that the pictures are not very clear and the technique is very expensive. To a large extent, PET is a scientific and experimental method. It is occasionally combined with MRI to produce clearer pictures.

SINGLE PHOTON EMISSION COMPUTED TOMOGRAPHY (SPECT)

To produce a SPECT picture, a substance that remains radioactive for some hours is injected into the blood stream. The blood carries the radioactive substance to all parts of the body. Areas of the body that use more blood receive more of the substance. The amount of radioactivity in the different parts of the body can be seen with a special camera.

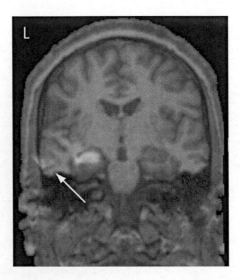

On a SPECT picture, areas with more radioactivity look bright and areas with less radioactivity look dark. The total amount of radioactive material given can be very small, since the special cameras are extremely sensitive.

The picture shows the result of a computer calculation in a person with seizures from the left temporal lobe. For this calculation, two SPECT pictures were taken: one between seizures and another during a seizure. Between seizures, a damaged area in the brain (like a scar) needs little blood and will show up dark on the SPECT picture. During a seizure, the area will show up bright on the SPECT picture because brain cells involved during a seizure use more blood than the rest of the brain. A computer can analyze the differences between both SPECT pictures and show where any abnormalities would be found on an MRI scan. The person shown in the picture could have an operation on the left side of the brain.

2.4 PROVOKING SEIZURES

MANY PEOPLE WITH EPILEPSY KNOW WHAT CAN TRIGGER THEIR SEIZURES

Many people know when they are at risk of having a seizure, but they cannot usually predict seizures with certainty or bring on seizures themselves. Sometimes seizures are most common in moments of relaxation after a period of strenuous exercise or concentration, especially if people are feeling a little worn out. Sometimes a loud noise or a particular smell can trigger seizures. Rarely, people have seizures whenever they do something complicated like playing a particular melody on a musical instrument. It always makes sense to try to find triggers for seizures, so that they can be avoided.

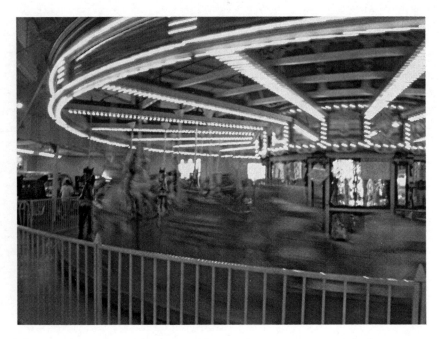

If, for instance, seizures are triggered by rapid movement, it may be best to try to avoid such movement (with permission from Gil Lhotka).

People who are prone to seizures when they have not had enough sleep can try to avoid getting up very early in the morning. However, it may not be possible to avoid triggers altogether, and there is a risk that people with epilepsy will avoid things that they enjoy (like meeting people or going out) although they are unlikely to bring on seizures.

SOMETIMES SEIZURES ARE PROVOKED IN THE HOSPITAL

In some people, seizures can be brought on by "provocation." Provocation is sometimes used during an EEG recording to bring out epileptic activity in the EEG. The most common methods of provocation are flashing light (photostimulation) and overbreathing (hyperventilation). Other methods include sleep deprivation or giving a smaller dose of epilepsy drugs.

Common Provocations of Seizures

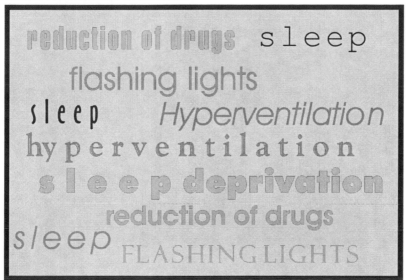

Provocation can cause epileptic seizures. However, most of the time, it only causes changes in the EEG that are typically seen in patients with epilepsy, and that suggest that someone has a tendency to have epileptic seizures. Flashing lights and hyperventilation can only provoke seizures in certain types of epilepsy. It is very easy, for instance, to bring on seizures in school age children with absence epilepsy by hyperventilation.

> Some people who know what triggers their seizures can avoid the trigger.

PEOPLE WHOSE SEIZURES ARE PROVOKED BY FLASHING LIGHT HAVE PHOTOSENSITIVE EPILEPSY

Asking someone to look at a flashing light can help to show whether he or she is at risk of having photosensitive epileptic seizures. However, photosensitivity is only found in a small number of people with epilepsy, and some people who have photosensitivity do not have seizures outside of possibly having seizures when exposed to flashing lights or other intense visual stimulation.

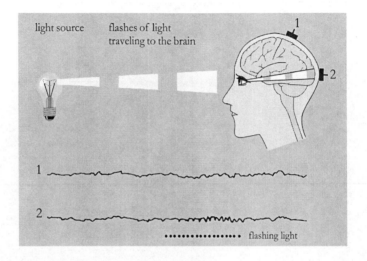

The flashes of light reach the back of the eye. They are translated into electrical impulses, which are passed on to the brain. Nerve cells on the surface of the brain are stimulated by each flash. In the picture, electrode (1) looks at an area of the brain not involved in seeing. Electrode (2) looks at the vision center. If the brain is not prone to photosensitive epileptic seizures, the flashes will cause no or only very small changes in the EEG. In the bottom right corner of the picture, each flash is marked by a black dot. The EEG was recorded from someone who is not at risk of photosensitive seizures. The waves under electrode (2), which are caused by the flashes, are only small. There is no photosensitivity.

IN SOME FORMS OF EPILEPSY, FLASHING LIGHTS CAUSE TYPICAL CHANGES IN THE EEG

Some types of EEG changes provoked by flashing lights suggest that a person has a tendency to develop epileptic activity or is at increased risk of developing epileptic seizures.

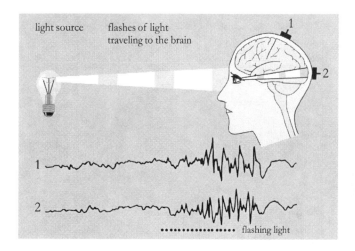

The EEG lines show waves triggered by the flashes of light. The waves get larger the longer the flashes continue. They can also be seen under electrode (1). This sort of EEG picture shows that the brain is prone to producing epileptic activity. There is increased photosensitivity. People who have EEG changes that are provoked by flashing lights often know that lights can bring on seizures and avoid situations where they may be at particular risk (for example in nightclubs, or if they sit close to the TV). However, 9 out of 10 people with epilepsy are not particularly sensitive to flashing light.

In people with increased photosensitivity, the EEG can show whether treatment is working.

DURING HYPERVENTILATION, PATIENTS BREATHE HARD WHILE THEY ARE RESTING

"Hyperventilation" means breathing more than necessary or breathing in and out deeply without doing any physical work at the same time. During hyperventilation, the EEG can show changes that suggest that someone is at risk of having epileptic seizures. The EEG changes are caused by a change in the amount of carbon dioxide (CO_2) in the blood. However, such changes are only seen in certain types of epilepsy.

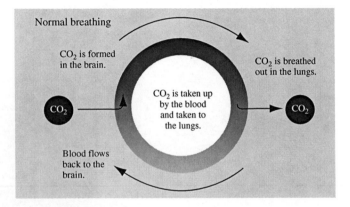

The body's organs make CO_2. During normal breathing, the CO_2 is taken up by the blood and breathed out by the lungs. The lungs breathe out as much CO_2 as the organs make. When the blood flows from the lungs to the organs of the body, it carries eight parts of CO_2. When it comes back to the lungs from the organs, it carries nine parts. Some of the CO_2 carried by the blood is not breathed out by the lungs but stays in the blood.

> Blood needs to carry the right amount of CO_2 to be able to fulfill many of its functions.

HYPERVENTILATION CAUSES THE CARBON DIOXIDE LEVELS IN THE BLOOD TO DROP

During hyperventilation, people breathe out more CO_2 than the body makes. This means that the amount of CO_2 that is stored in the blood goes down. This change in the blood causes changes in the brain that can be seen in the EEG. If typical changes are seen, they may suggest that someone is at higher risk of having epileptic seizures. However, hyperventilation changes the EEG only in particular types of epilepsy, for instance in absence epilepsy.

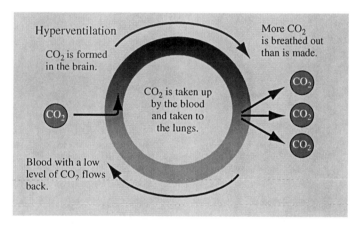

The picture shows that the blood changes when CO_2 levels are low. On the right side, more CO_2 is breathed out than is made by the body. This makes the blood more "alkaline." When the alkaline blood reaches the brain, it can change the working of nerve cells so that they produce epileptic activity. The blood can also become alkaline when people are sick or when they breathe hard because they are anxious or excited.

This picture shows how CO_2 in the blood drops during hyperventilation.

HARD WORK ALSO CAUSES DEEP BREATHING BUT DOES NOT PROVOKE SEIZURES

During physical work, the muscles have to work hard and use up more oxygen than when they are at rest. This means that they produce more CO_2. Breathing is increased, but only as much as is necessary to breathe out the extra CO_2. The CO_2 level in the arteries from the lungs to the brain does not change.

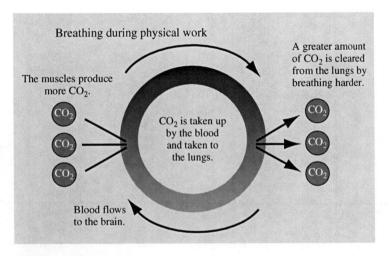

During physical activity, the level of CO_2 in the arteries does not change. The risk of an epileptic seizure is not increased.

Some people begin to breathe harder than necessary when they are anxious or stressed. When this happens, the muscles and organs of the body do not produce larger amounts of CO_2 than when they are at rest. Because of the overbreathing, the level of CO_2 in the blood carried to the brain changes and the blood becomes alkaline. In some people, alkaline blood can cause epileptic seizures.

In some people, hyperventilation can cause seizures.

LACK OF SLEEP CAN PROVOKE SEIZURES

In some people with epilepsy, lack of sleep (or "sleep deprivation") can bring on seizures. Sleep deprivation is sometimes used in the hospital to find out whether seizures are caused by epilepsy, or where in the brain they are coming from. To do this, the EEG is recorded after people have stayed awake through the night.

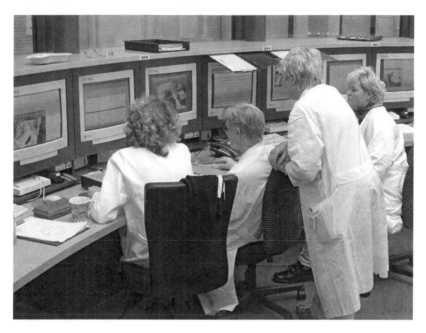

When seizures are provoked in the hospital, patients are often not just monitored with EEG but also with a video camera. The information from the EEG and the video recording of a seizure can show where the seizure started in the brain.

The fact that seizures can be provoked by lack of sleep shows how important it is for people with epilepsy to get enough sleep on a regular basis. Sometimes making sure that someone gets enough sleep stops seizures altogether. This means that medication changes or epilepsy surgery may not be necessary.

STRESS CAN INCREASE SEIZURE ACTIVITY

Stress and relaxation are at the opposite ends of a spectrum. Stress is the sum of biological reactions to a challenging situation. When someone is stressed, their heart activity and blood pressure increase and their muscular tension rises. Stress also has a range of effects on brain function.

Stress and relaxation are normal parts of life. However, some people experience many situations in life as stressful and are "stressed" much of the time.

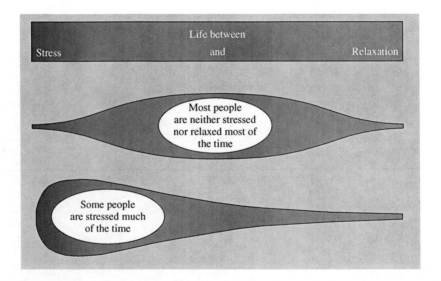

Stress can trigger seizure activity in several ways. It can increase the breathing rate and cause overbreathing or hyperventilation. Stress may also cause people to miss taking medication. Stress can cause hormonal changes such as an increase in the steroid hormone cortisol, which may influence seizure activity. Negative emotions related to stress, such as worry, anxiety, or depressed mood, may cause seizures.

Stress does not cause epilepsy to develop, but it can make seizures more likely.

People whose stress levels make their seizures worse can benefit from strategies that help them to deal more effectively with stress. Particularly stressful situations may be avoided, but some situations may not be avoidable. Relaxation techniques like yoga or tai chi can be learned. Exercise can also help people reduce stress. Recognizing one's limits and getting enough rest are also important. Lack of sleep can decrease the tolerance for stressful situations and increase the risk of seizures. If dealing with stress is a particularly severe problem, psychological treatments can help.

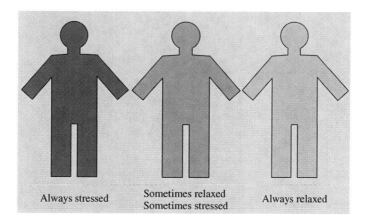

Always stressed   Sometimes relaxed   Always relaxed
                         Sometimes stressed

Stress can also be a problem for children. Parents should try to recognize what is stressful for their child.

Stress is also a problem for people with learning difficulties. Changes in daily routines can be particularly stressful, especially if the person with learning difficulties has little control over the changes and does not understand them. Caregivers need to be aware of this and explain any changes as much as possible.

If the stress is serious, it may be helpful to talk to a psychologist.

SEIZURES CAN BE PROVOKED BY TAKING CERTAIN DRUGS OR HERBS

Some illegal drugs, such as cocaine, can bring on seizures. More often, prescription medicines cause seizures as an unwanted side effect in the treatment of malaria, infections, and depression. These medicines provoke seizures more easily in people with epilepsy.

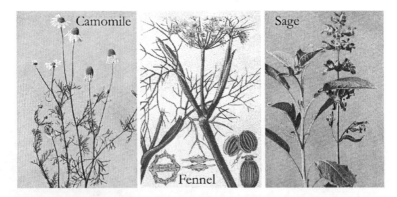

Some herbs that can make seizures worse are eucalyptus, fennel, hyssop, pennyroyal, rosemary, sage, savin, tansy, thuja, turpentine, and wormwood.

Some herbs can make seizures worse or weaken the effects of seizure medicines. For example, taking St. John's wort for more than a couple of weeks can lower the blood levels of the antiepileptic medicine carbamazepine. Long-term use of St. John's wort can also lower the effectiveness of birth control pills. Herbal medicines are widely sold for use in aromatherapy and massage, and some are taken orally. Although they are "natural," they are not necessarily harmless.

2.5 CAUSES OF EPILEPSY

EPILEPSY MAY BE CAUSED BY INHERITED AND ACQUIRED DAMAGE TO THE BRAIN

The risk of developing seizures is different for different people. This personal risk (or seizure susceptibility) can be high, moderate, or low. What determines someone's seizure susceptibility is not well known.

The EEG can provide some information about someone's seizure susceptibility when it shows many, a few, or no epileptic changes in the brain waves. However, the routine EEG cannot provide an exact measure of a person's seizure threshold or predict when a seizure will occur.

Some types of epilepsy (for instance primary generalized epilepsy) are predominantly caused by inherited traits. In most people, however, an inherited risk factor does not cause epilepsy on its own. Epilepsy only starts when something happens to the brain. The brain can be damaged or irritated in many ways.

COMMON CAUSES OF BRAIN DAMAGE

Brain damage can, for instance, consist of a scar caused by a head injury. Brain damage can also result from diseases affecting the brain.

Causes of Brain Damage:

- infection
- bleeding
- lack of oxygen
- brain injury in an accident
- problems with the body's metabolism
- tumor
- poor development of the brain
- interruption of the blood supply to the brain (stroke)
- abnormal aging (dementia)
- poisoning

Sometimes a combination of several types of brain damage causes epilepsy (for instance, an accident and lack of oxygen).

It is not completely understood how brain damage causes epileptic seizures.

BRAIN INJURY CAUSED BY AN ACCIDENT

Brain injuries can cause epileptic seizures within the first hour of having an accident, after months, or even years. More severe injuries are more likely to cause epilepsy.

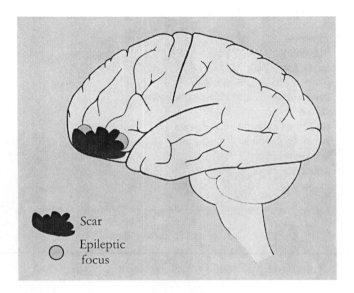

Scar

Epileptic
focus

Brain injuries that have caused bleeding into the brain are particularly likely to cause epilepsy. However, even very severe brain injuries cause epilepsy in only one-half of the people injured.

Example

Mrs. M. injured her brain in a car crash. She was unconscious for 3 days. Over the following weeks, she made a full recovery. The injury has scarred over. However, 1 year after the accident, she developed seizures caused by the brain tissue around the scar. She has to take antiepileptic medication.

DAMAGE CAUSED BY A TUMOR

A tumor causes pressure on the brain tissue around it. The brain cannot move out of the way because it is surrounded by the skull. This pressure may cause damage. It may also be responsible for headaches and for seizures. Sometimes seizures are the only symptom of a brain tumor.

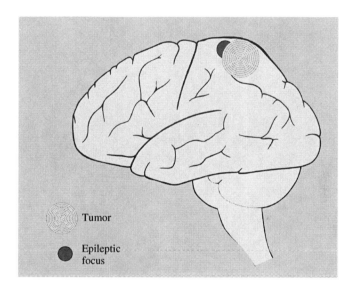

Tumor

Epileptic focus

It is possible that seizures will stop if the tumor can be removed by an operation.

Example

Mr. B. first had epileptic seizures 5 years ago, which stopped when antiepileptic medication was started. Although he continued to take his treatment, his seizures started again a few months ago. An MRI scan showed that the seizures were caused by a tumor. There is a good chance that the seizures will stop when the tumor has been removed.

DAMAGE CAUSED BY ALCOHOL

To suddenly stop taking alcohol after drinking heavily for weeks or months can cause alcohol withdrawal. Alcohol withdrawal commonly causes seizures. However, seizures may also be caused by smaller changes in the alcohol levels in the blood (for instance when people drink more or less than they normally do).

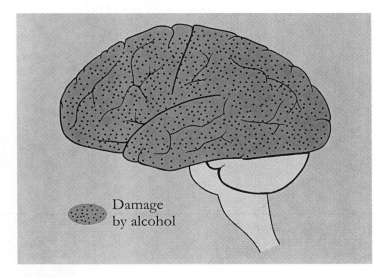

Lack of sleep increases the risk of seizures further. People who have seizures because of alcohol must stop drinking if they want to get better. If people drink large amounts of alcohol for many years, the alcohol can damage brain cells, so that epileptic seizures continue, even if they stop drinking alcohol. A high alcohol intake can also affect antiepileptic drug levels. This makes it difficult to treat epilepsy in people who continue to drink alcohol in excess.

Example

Mr. A. has had alcohol problems for 15 years. Although he has completed several alcohol withdrawal programs, he always starts drinking again. Over the years, alcohol has damaged his brain. From time to time, this damage causes epileptic seizures. The seizures could stop if Mr. A. would stop drinking.

DAMAGE CAUSED BY "FEBRILE SEIZURES"—SEIZURES RELATED TO HIGH TEMPERATURE

Fever sometimes causes seizures in babies. Occasionally, the seizures are so severe that children are taken to the hospital. In 9 out of 10 children, febrile seizures do not damage the brain. However, in particularly severe seizures, the combination of fever and seizures can damage the hippocampus in the temporal lobe of the brain.

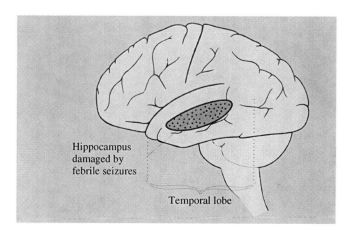

Hippocampus damaged by febrile seizures

Temporal lobe

It is not known how seizures can start with a fever, how fever and seizures damage the hippocampus, and how this damage can cause epilepsy.

Example

Mr. Z. had severe febrile seizures as a baby. Shortly after his 28th birthday, he developed a different type of seizure. Since that time, he has had frequent seizures, sometimes several in 1 day. The seizures always start with an odd sensation. Then Mr. Z. seems to clear his throat, fiddles with his clothes, and scratches around with his feet. It has not been possible to stop seizures with drugs. Three years after they first started, some seizures developed into tonic-clonic attacks. An MRI scan showed scarring of the hippocampus.

ABNORMAL DEVELOPMENT OF THE BRAIN IN THE WOMB

During the development of the brain in the womb, some cells act like tracks. They guide the nerve cells along the way from the place where they originate (at the bottom) to the place where they are meant to "live" and work (at the top in the outer layer called the cortex). This means that nerve cells have to travel (or "migrate") if the brain is to develop normally. Cells that do not reach their destination sometimes form small clumps (this abnormal development is called "microdysgenesis").

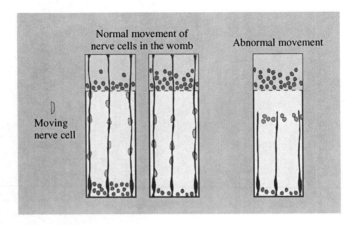

Clumps of cells that have not completed their migration are probably quite common. Only some of them cause epileptic seizures.

Example

Mrs. S. first had seizures at the age of 23. The seizures could not be stopped with drugs. She had many tests, and it was thought that her seizures could be stopped by an operation. After the operation, the seizures stopped but she still had to take antiepileptic drugs. The bit of brain that was removed at surgery was examined under the microscope. This examination showed microdysgenesis.

SEIZURES CAUSED BY PROBLEMS WITH THE BODY'S METABOLISM

The body constantly produces substances and breaks them down. All the different processes of production and breakdown together make up the body's "metabolism." Some problems with the metabolism can lead to seizures. For instance, people can develop epileptic seizures if there is not enough vitamin B6 in their diet. The seizures stop if they increase the vitamin B6 in their diet through food or if they take vitamin tablets. People who eat a healthy, varied diet are unlikely to develop problems because of a lack of vitamins.

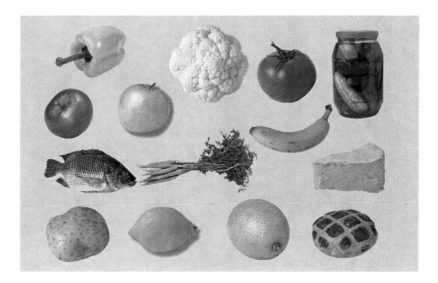

Most of us do not eat enough fruit and vegetables but eat too much fat, sugar, and protein.

Example

Three days after his birth, Joel's skin began to look yellow. Now that he was outside the womb, he needed fewer red blood cells. As his body was breaking down red blood cells, his liver produced a yellow dye. Joel had to spend a week under an ultraviolet lamp, which helped Joel's skin to break down the yellow dye more quickly. If the levels had risen any further in the blood, the dye could have caused epileptic seizures.

EPILEPTIC ACTIVITY CAN BE KINDLED

In animals, if the same area of the brain is irritated very slightly, for instance, with a low dose of electricity, nothing happens for the first days or weeks. However, after a few weeks, an epileptic focus develops. Repeated irritation can "kindle" epileptic activity. The irritation can be electrical, chemical, or physical. The irritation seems to increase seizure susceptibility—that is, the personal risk of seizures.

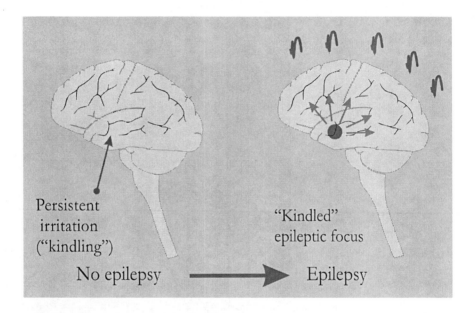

Persistent irritation ("kindling")

"Kindled" epileptic focus

No epilepsy ──────────▶ Epilepsy

At first, a kindled epileptic focus only produces epileptic activity whenever it is irritated. However, once this irritation has caused a number of epileptic seizures, epileptic activity can also be produced when the focus is not being irritated. It seems that the focus gets stronger and stronger. Because of this, it may be a good idea to treat seizures as early as possible with antiepileptic drugs. Every additional seizure could make it a little harder to stop epilepsy.

However, in many people with epilepsy, seizures do not seem to change over the years, which is why not all scientists believe this theory. This means that it is unlikely that the epileptic focus in these people has become any stronger.

BRAIN DAMAGE AND INHERITED FACTORS ADD UP

In the diagram, each column represents a different person. Each person has a different combination of brain damage and inherited risk of seizures (seizure susceptibility), symbolized by the two different shades. Seizures start when the combination of both is strong enough (that is, if the column is high enough). Person A, for instance, has inherited a low risk of seizures, but has acquired a large amount of brain damage. These factors add up and pass the threshold at which seizures start. Person C, however, has no seizures although his personal risk of seizure is much higher than that of person A.

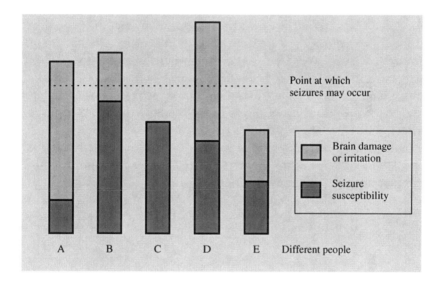

It is not understood what exactly seizure susceptibility is. It is, however, clear that an increased risk of seizures can be passed on to children from their parents. However, inherited factors often do not usually cause epilepsy on their own.

Sometimes EEG recordings of parents, brothers, or sisters of people with epilepsy also show epileptic activity, although they have never had an epileptic seizure. They may never develop seizures either.

THE RISK OF SEIZURES CHANGES AS PEOPLE GET OLDER

The risk of developing epilepsy is higher in the elderly than in younger adults. Conversely, a high body temperature may cause a seizure in a baby but not in a young otherwise healthy adult.

Any brain can produce epileptic activity and epileptic seizures under certain conditions. There are certain drugs, for instance, which can start seizures in anyone. Penicillin is one of these drugs. If people take very large amounts of this drug, they will develop seizures. Fifty years ago, when there were no other antibiotics 50 years ago, people with severe infections like meningitis or encephalitis were treated with such high doses of penicillin. Since only very low quantities of penicillin can pass from the blood to the brain, extremely large amounts of penicillin were used. The amount given was just below the level that could cause seizures. That is, people were treated with increasing amounts of penicillin until seizures appeared. Then the amount was slightly reduced in order not to trigger further epileptic seizures. The risks associated with a single seizure were smaller than the risks of meningitis or encephalitis. Today, we know more about the dosing of penicillin, so that seizures are hardly ever seen when penicillin is used to treat infections.

Penicillin is sometimes used in animal research of epilepsy. If a drop of penicillin solution is put onto the surface of the brain, an epileptic focus will develop within a few minutes.

Epileptic seizures can be provoked in anyone.

3

TREATING EPILEPSY

3.1 FIRST AID DURING A SEIZURE

FIRST AID DURING A TONIC-CLONIC SEIZURE

1. Stay calm

A tonic-clonic seizure is frightening to see, but it is not dangerous. Trying too hard to help or panicking will only make things worse. Watching the seizure calmly and trying to notice as many details as possible (especially how long it lasts) can help with further treatment.

2. Do not try to stop the seizure

The convulsion will stop by itself. Do not try to stop the movements of a seizure or to push anything in the mouth. It does not help and can cause injuries to the person having the seizure or the person who is trying to help.

3. Remove dangerous objects

The person having the seizure may have to be moved away from possible dangers (like traffic, if the seizure happens in the street). Other sources of danger (like furniture, sharp objects, or dangerous liquids) should be removed. Placing a cushion or some clothing under the head can prevent injuries.

4. After the seizure: Recovery position

If someone does not regain consciousness immediately after the seizure, it is best if they are placed in the recovery position on their side or on their stomach. People lying on their sides or stomach are less likely to choke on saliva. Any tight clothing around the neck should be loosened to allow people to breathe more easily.

5. After the seizure: Stay around

Often people are quite confused when they start to recover from an epileptic seizure. Therefore they should not be left alone. It is better to talk calmly to them and offer help. The confusion usually goes away in a few minutes.

6. Call an ambulance if . . .

. . . a seizure goes on for longer than 5 minutes or if there is a second seizure without full recovery from the first. If this happens, there is a risk of "status epilepticus" and a doctor should assess the situation as quickly as possible.

You may also have to call an ambulance if the seizure has caused an injury.

HELPING SOMEONE DURING A COMPLEX PARTIAL SEIZURE

It is usually not possible to prevent a seizure from developing fully or to stop a seizure once it has started. While the seizure goes on, dangerous objects (for instance, a burning candle) should be placed well out of reach. After the seizure, people may be confused for 10 or 20 minutes. During this time they should not be left alone. They should be watched to make sure that they do not injure themselves.

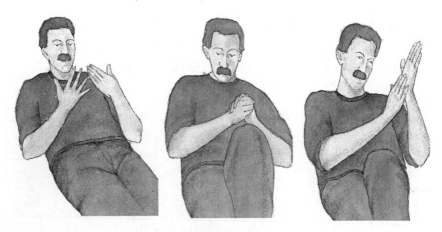

A single complex partial seizure is over after a few minutes. However, one seizure may be followed by another so quickly that the person does not "wake up" fully between attacks. This condition is called "complex partial status epilepticus" (or "non-convulsive status epilepticus"). It is not life-threatening but may need to be treated with medication. Usually patients with complex partial status have to go to the hospital.

Complex partial status epilepticus has to be treated by a doctor.

SEIZURES RELATED TO FEVER CAN BE PREVENTED
BY BRINGING DOWN HIGH TEMPERATURES

Babies and young children can develop a fever very quickly. Sometimes this causes "febrile seizures." Severe febrile seizures can occasionally cause epilepsy many years later. Febrile seizures are severe when they last for more than 15 minutes or if one seizure follows on immediately from another. Febrile seizures are not epilepsy because they are seizures that are "provoked" by fever.

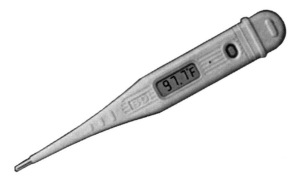

Because of the risk that febrile seizures could cause epilepsy in later life, temperatures should not be allowed to rise too highly or quickly in children under 5. Parents usually learn to recognize when their child has a fever.

If the child shows signs of fever, the temperature should be measured. In children who have already had a febrile convulsion in the past, temperatures above 102 degrees Fahrenheit (39 degrees Centigrade) should be treated with medicine as directed by a doctor.

Parents can also soak towels in cold water and wrap them around the calves of the child. This has to be repeated every few minutes. The thermometer will show whether the temperature has gone down.

High temperatures in small children with previous febrile seizures should be brought down to prevent further febrile seizures.

HOW TO GET THE RIGHT KIND OF HELP

People with epilepsy often find themselves in a hospital after a seizure although they have recovered fully and feel well again. Bystanders have called an ambulance because they did not know what else to do. This would be different if people knew more about epilepsy.

- Talk to the people around you (colleagues, neighbors) about your seizures. If you do not want to use the word "epilepsy," you could always tell them about your "blackouts" or "seizures."
- Try to explain as clearly as possible what exactly happens during your seizures and how long they go on for.
- Explain that seizures are not usually dangerous and generally stop by themselves.
- Tell people what you would like them to do (and what you would like them not to do) when you have a seizure.

It can be difficult to talk to people in this way. It is important to pick a good time for such a talk. However, you will find that people are much less anxious and insecure once you have told them about your seizures and they know what to do if you have one.

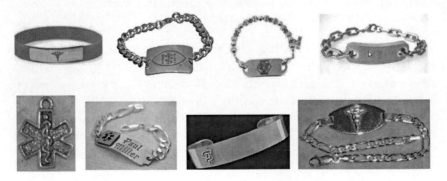

Several types of medical bracelets are available.

An emergency card, bracelet, or locket can also help to inform people who may find you during a seizure.

3.2 TREATMENT WITH DRUGS

DRUGS CAN STOP SEIZURES—THEY ARE CALLED ANTIEPILEPTIC DRUGS

The aim of using antiepileptic drugs is to stop seizures. This cannot always be achieved; sometimes, taking antiepileptic drugs only means that there are fewer seizures.

In some people, the tendency to have seizures eventually goes away and drugs can be stopped under the doctor's supervision. Often, however, antiepileptic treatment has to be taken for the long term, for years or even for life. It is important that the right dose of the drugs is taken every day. People who do not take their antiepileptic drugs regularly do not protect themselves well against seizures. Taking antiepileptic drugs on and off may even cause seizures to worsen.

Although antiepileptic drugs do not cure epilepsy, they protect the brain against seizures. This protection can be compared to the safety features of a car. An airbag cannot stop an accident but it can protect the driver of the car from injury.

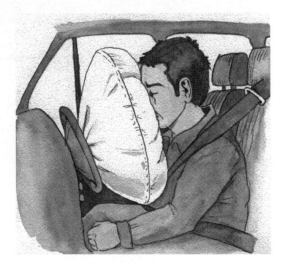

An airbag protects against injuries like antiepileptic drugs can prevent seizures. Airbags do not stop accidents, just as antiepileptic drugs do not cure epilepsy.

> Antiepileptic drugs can stop seizures; however, they do not cure epilepsy.

SOMETIMES DRUGS ARE NO LONGER NEEDED

Epilepsy can go away in some cases when seizures have been stopped for several years by antiepileptic drugs. The only way to know for sure, however, is to taper off the drugs very slowly, often over weeks or months. If the seizures do not come back, the epilepsy has gone. But in some cases, lowering the dose of antiepileptic drugs can cause epileptic seizures to return. It is not possible to know in advance of stopping medications whether someone will or will not have recurrent seizures. Sometimes it is hard to regain control of seizures once the medications are restarted. Antiepileptic drugs should therefore be tapered off only under medical supervision.

CAN THE BRAIN FORGET HOW TO PRODUCE SEIZURES?

We do not fully understand how people learn and how they forget. However, it sometimes seems as if the brain can forget how to produce epileptic activity.

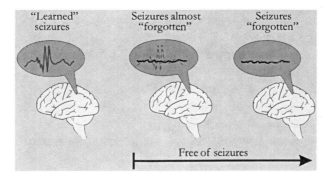

Drugs may help the brain to forget by stopping seizures. This sort of healing process occurs in some types of epilepsy but is extremely rare in others.

> **Any change in the dose of an antiepileptic drug should be done under the direction of a specialist.**

REASONS FOR USING ANTIEPILEPTIC DRUGS

Most people with epilepsy can become free of seizures if they take antiepileptic drugs. There are many reasons why it may be important for people to be free of seizures. Which reasons are most important will depend on individual circumstances. Before drugs are started, it is best to talk about this with a doctor.

- Seizures can cause injuries.
- Seizures can cause problems at work and at home, and they can interfere with hobbies or recreational activities.
- Convulsions lasting longer than 30 minutes (status epilepticus) can potentially cause permanent brain damage.
- Drug treatment can stop focal seizures from developing into generalized seizures.
- There may be problems with memory and concentration for several hours after a seizure. This can cause problems at school or at work.
- People who have seizures cannot take part in certain sports (for instance, deep-sea diving).
- People who have active epileptic seizures are usually not allowed to drive a car.
- If seizures occur in the bath or while swimming, they can possibly cause drowning.
- The risk of sudden unexpected death is higher when there are active seizures than when someone's seizures are fully controlled by medication.
- Epilepsy will sometimes not return after it has been controlled with drugs.

REASONS AGAINST USING ANTIEPILEPTIC DRUGS

People who have very mild or infrequent seizures and people with epilepsy whose seizures have not got better at all with medication should discuss the pros and cons of taking antiepileptic drugs with their doctors. It is difficult to measure how mild or severe epilepsy is. Much depends on the circumstances of the person having the seizures.

Here are some examples of mild epilepsy: if there has been one tonic-clonic seizure from sleep per year for many years, or if there is twitching of the muscles of the left hand for a few minutes every week but no other seizures.

Further considerations for deciding whether to take antiepileptic drugs:

- Antiepileptic drugs can cause side effects.
- Antiepileptic drugs taken in pregnancy may increase the risk of malformations in the child.
- Antiepileptic drugs can change the effects of other medications.

Drug treatment can be difficult and may require a lot of patience to achieve just the right medicine and dosage. Often, the difficulties cannot be foreseen. For instance, an antiepileptic drug may not be effective even though it works well in other people with a similar type of epilepsy.

WHEN DRUGS ARE STARTED AND WHEN THEY ARE STOPPED

Antiepileptic drug treatment should be considered when someone has had their first epileptic seizure. Depending on the particular circumstances, the risk of further seizures ranges from 20 to 80 percent. People with a low risk of seizure recurrence may decide with their physician to hold off medication until further seizures have proven that they really need to take antiepileptic drugs. The risk of further seizures is higher when the neurological examination, a brain scan, or brainwave recording (EEG) is abnormal.

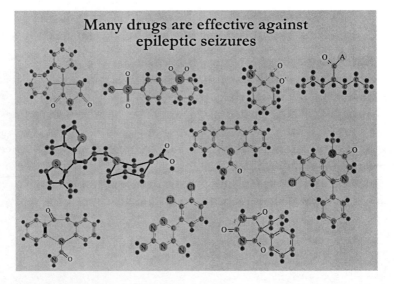

Many drugs are effective against epileptic seizures

Goals of treatment with drugs: Control of seizures, minimal side effects, and optimal quality of life.

If no more seizures have occurred during 1, 2, or 3 years, the possibility of stopping medication may be discussed with a doctor. Drugs should not be stopped suddenly—they need to be tapered off gradually to minimize the risk of seizures getting worse.

When thinking about whether to stop antiepileptic drugs, people need to consider the impact that further seizures would have on their lives. This may include the loss of their driving license and problems at their workplace or with their leisure interests. The risk of seizures coming back after stopping antiepileptic drugs ranges from 5 to 90 percent. The risk is higher if there is a history of generalized tonic-clonic or myoclonic seizures, if more than one drug was needed to control seizures, or if there are abnormalities on a brain scan or EEG.

SEIZURES ARE STOPPED BY THE ACTIVE INGREDIENT IN A DRUG

The name of the active ingredient (also called "generic name") is printed on the box of tablets. Sometimes drugs also have a "brand name." Brand names are made up by the pharmaceutical companies that produce the tablets. Sometimes the same active ingredient is sold under different brand names. For instance, Tegretol and Carbatrol both contain the active ingredient carbamazepine.

TABLETS DO NOT JUST CONTAIN THE ACTIVE INGREDIENT

Pharmaceutical companies often use secret chemical processes to make the tablets they sell. They may, for instance, add substances that cause the active ingredient to be released in the small bowel rather than the stomach. This makes each tablet work longer.

Because of such differences, tablets containing the same active ingredient can have different effects if they are made by different companies. This means that there may be problems switching over, for example, from one type of carbamazepine to another. Because of this, a drug that is working should only be changed in an emergency or after careful consideration.

TREATMENT WITH DRUGS MAY BE DIFFICULT AND DOES NOT ALWAYS WORK

Research has shown which drugs work for epilepsy. However, it is never clear which drug will work best in a particular person. About one-half of people with epilepsy become free of seizures with the first drug they try.

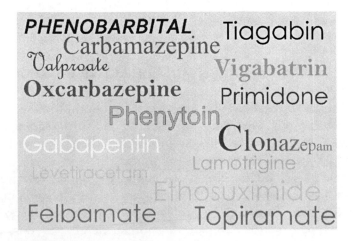

Researched drugs that work for people with epilepsy.

As a rule of thumb, larger doses of drugs work better than smaller doses. On the other hand, larger doses may cause more side effects. Because of this, it is best to use the lowest antiepileptic drug dose that stops seizures. It can sometimes take months or years to find the right drug and the right dose. It is important that doctors and people with epilepsy remain patient in their search for the best treatment.

It is never certain in advance of trying whether the drug of first choice will have any useful effect.

THE RIGHT DRUG HAS TO BE FOUND—SOMETIMES SEVERAL DRUGS HAVE TO BE TRIED

When treatment is started for epilepsy, it is never certain in advance of trying that the first drug chosen will actually work. However, the chance of stopping seizures is highest with the first type of treatment. If seizures continue, the dose is increased. If a drug causes unpleasant side effects or if it does not have enough of an effect on seizures, a different drug is tried. Usually, it takes some time to switch from one drug to another.

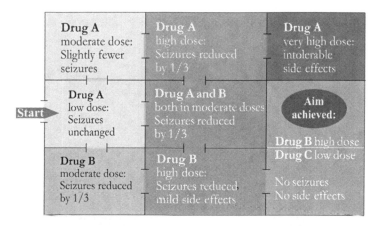

For a doctor, starting epilepsy treatment is like entering a house he or she has not been in before. The goal is to stop all seizures, which might be possible immediately after stepping into the house. But he or she may have to make their way through several rooms to the back of the house, and it may not be possible to achieve the goal at all. The example shows a type of epilepsy that usually gets better with drug A or B.

ANTIEPILEPTIC DRUGS HAVE TO GET INTO THE BRAIN

Once a tablet has been swallowed, it travels through the stomach into the bowels. This is where most tablets are dissolved and where the active ingredients are set free. These ingredients are taken up by the blood in the wall of the bowels and carried throughout the whole body by the bloodstream. In this way, drugs also reach the brain, where they can stop seizures.

Drugs may not get into the brain when people are sick or when they have diarrhea. If tablets are vomited up or if the walls of the bowels cannot take up the drug, there is a higher risk of seizures.

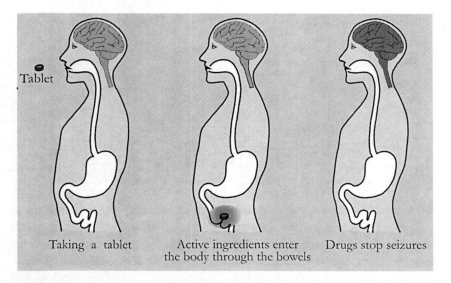

Taking a tablet   Active ingredients enter   Drugs stop seizures
                         the body through the bowels

The strength of treatment does not depend on the number of tablets but on the dose of the drug and the amount of the drug that has entered the body. A single tablet containing 500 mg of a drug is stronger than three tablets of the same drug each containing 100 mg.

The amount (or concentration) of a drug in the body can be measured with blood tests.

MOST DRUGS ARE BROKEN DOWN BY THE LIVER

The picture shows how the heart pumps blood into the brain and into the walls of the bowels. A tablet is dissolving in the bowels. The blood in the picture flows from the right to the left, past the tablet. It takes up the active ingredient (shown by the shading of the blood). Some of the drug never reaches the brain: It is carried through the liver and broken down there. The rest is carried past the liver to the heart. From there, it is pumped to the brain, where it can stop seizures.

THE DRUG CONCENTRATION IN THE BLOOD CHANGES

The amount of a drug in the blood is greatest in the bowels where the tablets have dissolved. The amount is smaller in the blood that arrives from the bowels in the heart because some of the drug has been broken down and passed out of the body by the liver.

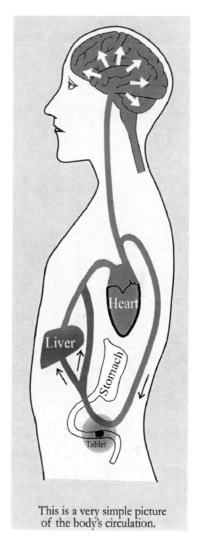

This is a very simple picture of the body's circulation.

> **Drugs have to be taken every day because they are constantly cleared by the body.**

EACH TABLET STOPS SEIZURES FOR ONLY A SHORT TIME

Tablets do not work straightaway. It usually takes several hours before they are dissolved in the bowels, taken up by the blood, and work in the brain. One single tablet is rarely enough to stop the brain from producing epileptic seizures.

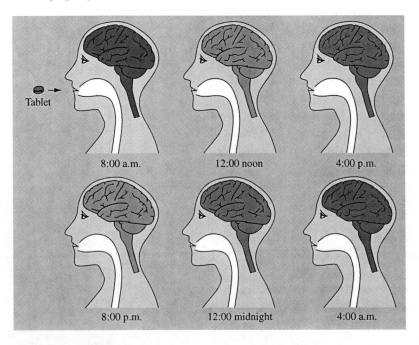

The picture shows how the high risk of a seizure (light gray) is lowered for a short time by the antiepileptic drug (shown in dark gray). In this example, the tablet offers good protection for about 8 hours. It begins to work only a few hours after the tablet has been swallowed because it takes time for the body to take up the active ingredients and to deliver them to the brain. The effect of the drug wears off because the body breaks it down and clears it.

Some antiepileptic drugs have to be taken several times a day.

DRUGS HAVE TO BE TAKEN REGULARLY SO THAT THEY CAN PROTECT AGAINST SEIZURES

To achieve protection against seizures around the clock, the same amount of a drug has to be fed into the body as is broken down and passed out. This sort of balance is called "steady state."

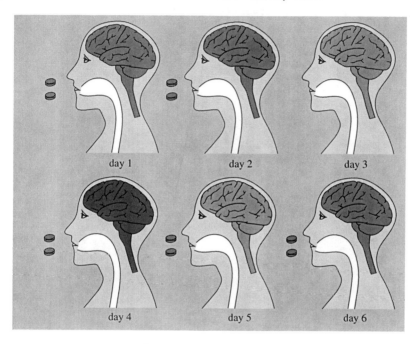

If tablets are taken regularly (for instance, as two tablets once a day) and at the right dose, the amount of the drug that enters the body is the same as the amount that passes out of it. The concentration of the drug in the brain (dark gray) will then remain steady. If tablets are forgotten or drugs are not taken up by the bloodstream because of vomiting or diarrhea, the risk of seizures (black) goes up as on days 3, 4, and 5 in the picture.

Tablets have to be taken every day because it is not known when seizures could happen.

A PILLBOX CAN MAKE IT EASIER TO TAKE TABLETS REGULARLY EVERY DAY

If tablets are not taken regularly, the brain is not always protected against seizures. Taking tablets on and off can even make epilepsy worse. Pillboxes can help people to remember to take their tablets every day. These boxes can hold tablets for a whole week.

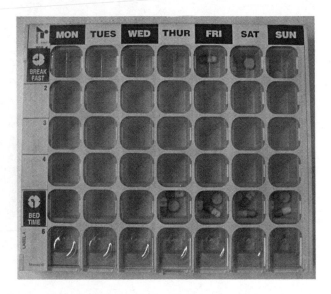

This is a picture of a pillbox for 1 week. There are several compartments for each day, for the morning, lunchtime, afternoon, and so forth. The box can be filled once a week. Each compartment can be opened separately with a slider. The pillbox in the picture has been used up to Thursday afternoon. The Thursday morning tablets have been taken. The owner of the box takes three tablets at nighttime.

People with epilepsy who have become free of seizures through antiepileptic drugs should not risk having more seizures by not taking their tablets regularly. As drugs are broken down and cleared by the body all the time, they have to be taken on a regular basis, as prescribed by the physician.

3.3 ANTIEPILEPTIC DRUGS

ANTIEPILEPTIC DRUGS (MEDICINES) ACT ON NERVE CELLS IN THE BRAIN

Many of the effects that drugs have on nerve cells are known. However, it is often not clear which one of the effects (or which combination of effects) stops seizures. At the moment, only three of four people with epilepsy can be treated successfully with the drugs available. This means that there is a great need for new antiepileptic drugs.

New drugs are often discovered in the way in which Christopher Columbus discovered America over 500 years ago. Unlike his contemporaries, he thought that the world was not flat but round. So he sailed off to the west to find a new sea route to India. He found America by accident.

Most antiepileptic drugs were also discovered by chance. For instance, 40 years ago, scientists were looking for new drugs for heart conditions. They produced chemical substances that seemed likely to have effects on the heart. However, the substances they had made could not be dissolved in water. Therefore, they could not have reached the heart through the blood. To help dissolve the drugs in water, they were mixed with a substance called dipropylacetate. As it happened, the new drugs had no effects on the heart. However, it was

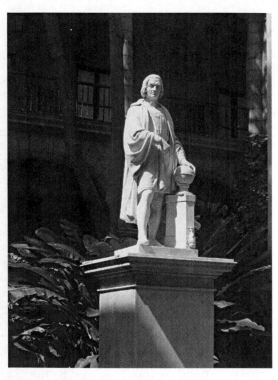

With permission from Paul W. Peters

noted by chance that they stopped epileptic seizures. Sometime later, the scientists realized that it was not the useless heart drugs that were stopping seizures but the dipropylacetate. Today this substance is used as valproate.

DRUGS CAN STOP THE DEVELOPMENT OF EPILEPTIC ACTIVITY IN THE BRAIN

Seizures are caused by abnormal electrical activity in nerve cells. In the picture, a nerve cell producing such epileptic activity is marked in a darker shade. Research is beginning to explain how epileptic activity develops. Little channels in the wall of the nerve cell play an important role. In particular, channels specializing in the transport of calcium ions and potassium ions are responsible for the development of epileptic activity.

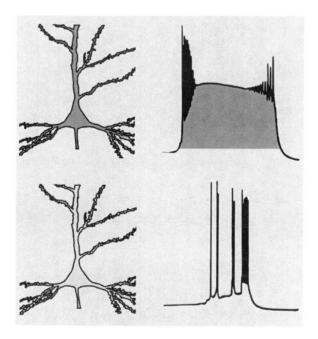

Top: Nerve cell producing epileptic activity while being flooded with calcium ions. Bottom: Treated nerve cell, protected from being overwhelmed by calcium ions.

Many antiepileptic drugs have an effect on the channels in the cell wall. Drugs that hold up the flow of calcium ions into the cell can stop epileptic activity and seizures. Epileptic activity can also be stopped by blocking the flow of sodium ions or by increasing the flow of potassium ions into cells. Several of the antiepileptic drugs used today work in this way.

DRUGS CAN STOP THE SPREAD OF EPILEPTIC ACTIVITY IN THE BRAIN

An epileptic focus is an area of the brain that produces epileptic activity. In the picture, the focus is the inner semicircle. The brain surrounds such a focus with a rim of cells whose job it is to stop the spread of epileptic activity to the rest of the brain.

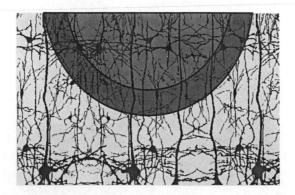

Epileptic focus with rim of brain cells trying to stop the spread of epileptic activity.

This rim acts like a dam that stops epileptic activity from spilling over to other brain areas. Antiepileptic drugs can strengthen this rim and help protect the rest of brain.

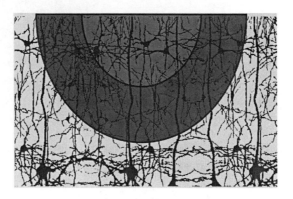

A drug has strengthened the rim around an epileptic focus.

Some drugs do not stop the production of epileptic activity (which can still be seen in the EEG), but they do stop the spread of this activity. They can do this by strengthening the brain's defenses against epileptic activity.

DRUGS CAN STOP BRAIN CELLS FROM FALLING IN STEP WITH ONE ANOTHER

The epileptic signals that are picked up in the EEG and that cause the twitching of muscles during a seizure are produced by groups of nerve cells firing off electrical activity in step with one another (or synchronously). This sort of "synchronicity" is typical of epileptic activity and means that many nerve cells are firing at the same time. The picture shows a group of nerve cells producing abnormally synchronous epileptic activity.

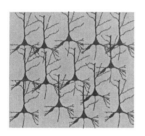
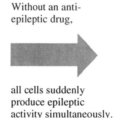
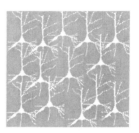

Without an antiepileptic drug,

all cells suddenly produce epileptic activity simultaneously.

Seizures can be prevented by stopping groups of brain cells from discharging electrical activity at the same time.

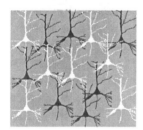
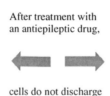
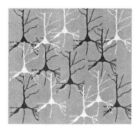

After treatment with an antiepileptic drug,

cells do not discharge at the same time.

Several epilepsy drugs can affect groups of nerve cells in this way. They act by different chemical means and may work on different centers in the brain.

CARBAMAZEPINE (CBZ)

Carbamazepine (CBZ) is one of the most commonly used antiepileptic medicines. CBZ is the name of the active substance (the generic name). CBZ is contained in the brands Carbatol, Epitol, Tegretol, and Tegretol XR (which releases carbamazepine more slowly than Tegretol). Such tablets release CBZ more slowly in the body.

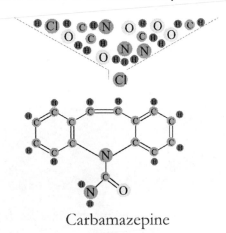

Carbamazepine

The drug is made up of:

C : Carbon

H : Hydrogen

N : Nitrogen

O : Oxygen

Like most other drugs, CBZ is broken down and passed out by the body all the time. Tablets therefore have to be taken at least twice a day.

Carbamazepine dissolves in the intestine and is taken up by the bloodstream. It is broken down in the liver. If seizures were first stopped by carbamazepine and then started again, the amount of CBZ in the body may have dropped. The amount of CBZ in the body can be measured with a blood test. Sometimes a higher dose can stop seizures again. In other cases, a different antiepileptic drug or a combination of drugs would be better.

Carbamazepine is often used as the first antiepileptic drug. It can stop many types of seizures. However, one can never be certain in advance which dose will stop the seizures. As with other antiepileptic drugs, the right dose has to be found for everyone. People who have never been treated with antiepileptic drugs before often become free of seizures with a relatively low dose of CBZ.

CBZ does not work for absence seizures and may even make them worse.

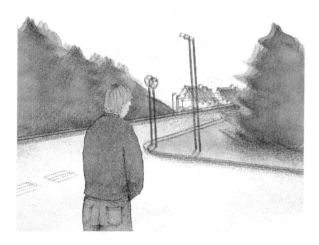

Occasionally, carbamazepine causes side effects. Some people have an allergic reaction to it. Usually this causes a skin rash. Most people who are allergic to CBZ have to stop taking it.

Double or blurred vision is a common side effect of CBZ. It is annoying but not dangerous unless people are doing something for which they need clear vision. The double vision always improves when the amount of CBZ is reduced. However, changes of antiepileptic drug dosages should always be discussed with a doctor first.

CBZ causes the liver to break down other drugs more quickly. This weakens the effects of the oral contraceptive pill. People on CBZ who want to stay on oral contraceptives may have to take a higher dose of the contraceptive pill. They may also consider using other forms of contraception like condoms or a diaphragm.

PHENYTOIN (PHT)

Phenytoin has been used as a treatment for epileptic seizures for some 70 years. Phenytoin is the name of the active ingredient contained in the registered brands Dilantin and Phenytek. Apart from PHT tablets, capsules, and syrup, there are also solutions of PHT that can be injected into a vein. The capsules or tablets contain 30, 50, 100, 200, or 300 mg of PHT. The solution is mostly used in the hospital as a treatment for status epilepticus.

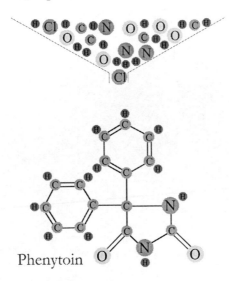

Phenytoin

The drug is made up of:

C : Carbon
H : Hydrogen
N : Nitrogen
O : Oxygen

Phenytoin is broken down and passed out of the body by the liver. To replace the amount passed out of the body it has to be taken at least once a day.

Phenytoin is only taken up slowly from the intestine. Because of this, the level of PHT rises gradually over 6 hours after a tablet has been taken. After 6 hours the amount of PHT begins to fall and, after around 30 hours, only half the amount of PHT is left in the body. Given that it stays in the body for such a long time, it is often possible to take the whole amount of PHT needed to protect the brain for the day in a single dose.

Phenytoin is used for generalized or focal seizures. It does not tend to work very well for seizures in babies or toddlers. Many people get no side effects from PHT. However, as with other drugs against seizures, side effects are more likely when people take high doses of PHT. High levels of PHT can cause nausea, vomiting, double vision, dizziness, and trembling of the hands.

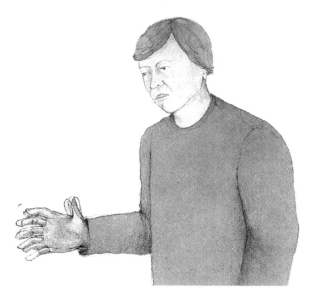

Sometimes, PHT can affect the way people look, for example it can cause the gums to grow thicker. Such thickening of the gums (or gum "hypertrophy") can be corrected. It can also be prevented to some extent by taking good care of the teeth. Rarely, PHT can cause an increase of body hair or brown patches on the skin.

PHT can reduce the effect of other drugs. Drugs that work less well when people also take PHT include blood thinners and the oral contraceptive pill. Women who need to take PHT and who also want to take the contraceptive pill may need to take a higher dose of the contraceptive.

VALPROATE (VPA)

Valproate or valproic acid (VPA) is the active ingredient in the brands Depakene, Depacon, Depakote, and Depakote ER. VPA is also available as a syrup and a solution for injection into a vein.

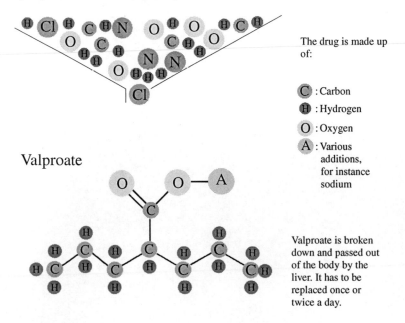

The drug is made up of:

C : Carbon

H : Hydrogen

O : Oxygen

A : Various additions, for instance sodium

Valproate

Valproate is broken down and passed out of the body by the liver. It has to be replaced once or twice a day.

Normally, drugs are stronger if their amount in the body is greater. When treatment with VPA is started, the total amount of VPA in the body increases over some days. Eventually, the amount of VPA taken and the amount passed out every day are in balance. Although the amount of VPA in the body does not increase after this, its effectiveness against seizures continues to grow stronger for some time.

Valproate is often used to stop generalized seizures but it also works for focal seizures. VPA is particularly useful for stopping absence and myoclonic seizures. Seizures that are provoked by flashing light and other primary generalized seizures can also be treated with VPA.

VPA can cause stomach pain and sickness. This can be reduced by using forms of VPA that dissolve slowly in the intestine (Depakote and Depakote ER). Most side effects caused by valproate occur soon after starting the treatment and pass after a while. Valproate can reduce the ability of the blood to seal off small wounds. Some people who have this problem can bruise easily or can have nose-bleeds. People who take VPA should warn a surgeon or a dentist about this before they have an operation.

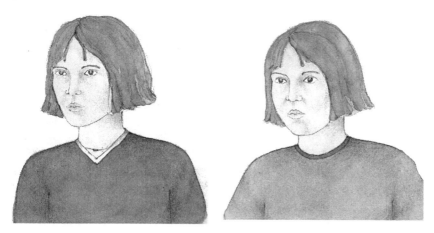

Valproate can also affect people's looks. It can, for instance, cause hair loss. Although the hair usually grows back if VPA is stopped, it sometimes is more crinkly and has a slightly different color from the original hair. VPA can also cause weight gain. This means that people taking VPA should keep an eye on their weight. Women who take valproate can develop irregular periods. Occasionally, VPA makes acne worse. Very rarely, VPA causes severe damage to the liver or pancreas.

PHENOBARBITAL (PB)

Phenobarbital belongs to a group of drugs called barbiturates. Phenobarbital is also made by the body when it breaks down primidone, another drug used to treat seizures. PB is contained in the brand Luminal. Apart from tablets, there is a PB syrup and a solution that can be injected into veins or muscles. Barbiturates have been used to treat seizures for about 90 years. In the past, they were also used as sleeping tablets. They are still given today to put people to sleep for operations.

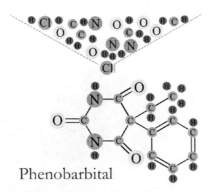

Phenobarbital

The drug is made up of:

C : Carbon
H : Hydrogen
O : Oxygen
N : Nitrogen

Phenobarbital is broken down by the body all the time and has to be replaced at least once a day.

Phenobarbital is taken up only slowly in the intestines. It is also broken down and passed out of the body at a slow rate. This means that it is possible to replace the whole amount of PB needed for the day in a single dose. If PB is started at such a replacement or "maintenance" dose, it takes 3 weeks for the drug level to build up in the body. If PB has to be started more quickly, it can be introduced with a higher "loading" dose, which is then lowered to the normal daily dose after a few days. If PB is stopped, it takes a long time until the drug has passed completely out of the body. PB can reduce the effect of the oral contraceptive pill and it can cause a lack of vitamin D, which can weaken the bones.

Phenobarbital is an effective treatment for generalized and focal seizures. It can also be used in status epilepticus. It is sometimes used in small children to prevent seizures with high temperature (febrile convulsions). PB can make absence seizures worse.

The main side effect of PB is tiredness. In children, PB sometimes causes the opposite effect—overactivity and unusual irritability. PB can also cause difficulties with concentration, and it may increase reaction time. This can cause problems if people have to react quickly in traffic or if they operate dangerous machinery.

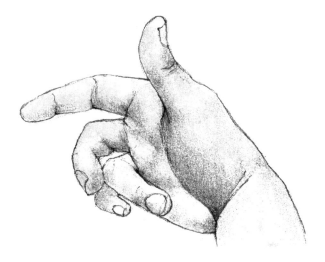

Dupuytren contracture.

People who have taken phenobarbital for many years sometimes develop a condition called "polyfibromatosis." There is thickening of the connective tissue, particularly in the hands. The tendons become thicker and shorter, and it becomes increasingly difficult for people to stretch their fingers (called Dupuytren contracture). The shoulders may be affected, too.

PB should never be stopped suddenly. This can cause "withdrawal" seizures.

BENZODIAZEPINES (BDZS)

Benzodiazepines (BDZs) are a group of drugs. A number of BDZs are used to treat seizures: clobazam, clonazepam, clorazepate, diazepam, lorazepam, and nitrazepam. The following brands contain BDZs: Ativan, Diastat, Diazepam Intensol, Dizac, Klonopin, Lorazepam Intensol, Serax, Tranxene-SD, Valium, Frisium, Mogadon, and Tranxene (some of these are used in Canada). BDZs can be given as tablets, and some preparations can be injected into a vein, the nose, mouth, or into the rectum. BDZs are not only used in the treatment of epileptic seizures. They also have many other uses, for instance as sleeping tablets and to help in the treatment of anxiety.

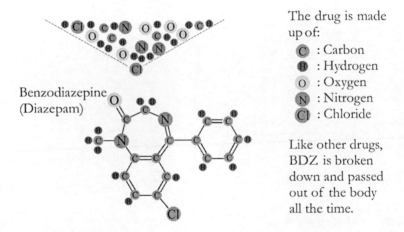

Benzodiazepine
(Diazepam)

The drug is made up of:

C : Carbon
H : Hydrogen
O : Oxygen
N : Nitrogen
Cl : Chloride

Like other drugs, BDZ is broken down and passed out of the body all the time.

BDZs act very quickly and can be injected into a vein or inserted into the rectum during a flurry of seizures or status epilepticus.

Benzodiazepines work very well for most types of seizures. They can sometimes block seizures that were not stopped by carbamazepine or phenytoin. Unfortunately, the effect of BDZs can wear off. When this has happened, they usually work again once they have not been taken for a few weeks. Because of these problems, BDZs are rarely used in the long-term treatment of seizures. However, they are very useful for status epilepticus, or in people who have seizures only at particular times, for instance women who have seizures only around their menstrual period.

The main side effect of BDZs is tiredness and poor concentration. BDZs can affect reaction time and may therefore cause problems when people have to react quickly in traffic or when they operate dangerous machines. In children, BDZs can sometimes cause irritability and hyperactivity.

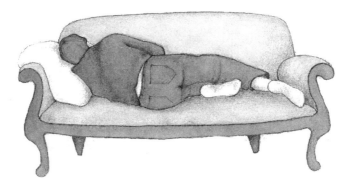

If BDZs are taken for some time, people can become addicted to them. The main symptom of such an addiction is that people who suddenly stop their BDZs feel very anxious. They can also develop muscle cramps or the kinds of symptoms that heavy drinkers have if they stop alcohol suddenly. Such withdrawal symptoms, however, are not common in patients who take BDZs for epilepsy. One reason for this is that the BDZs doses used to treat seizures are relatively small.

LAMOTRIGINE (LTG)

Lamotrigine has been used to treat seizures for about 20 years. Lamotrigine is contained in the brand Lamictal. Several studies have shown that LTG is an effective treatment for seizures.

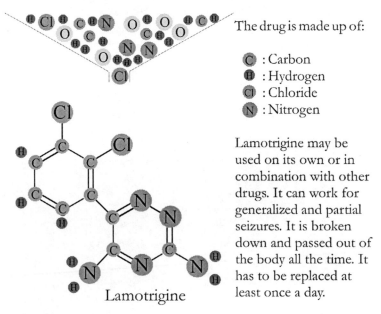

The drug is made up of:

C : Carbon
H : Hydrogen
Cl : Chloride
N : Nitrogen

Lamotrigine may be used on its own or in combination with other drugs. It can work for generalized and partial seizures. It is broken down and passed out of the body all the time. It has to be replaced at least once a day.

Lamotrigine

Lamotrigine has a similar effect on seizures as phenytoin and carbamazepine.

Lamotrigine can be used on its own (as "monotherapy") or in combination with other drugs. It can stop seizures in many types of epilepsy.

As a positive side effect, LTG sometimes improves the mood of people who are feeling depressed. LTG reduces the effectiveness of the oral contraceptive pill slightly. This does not necessarily mean that the contraceptive pill would be ineffective. Women taking LTG should discuss the best method of contraception with their doctor. The oral contraceptive pill can also reduce the level of LTG in the blood by up to 30 percent. This means that women taking the contraceptive pill may need to take higher doses of LTG.

Lamotrigine causes side effects in fewer people than carbamazepine. In higher doses, it can cause weakness, tiredness, and double vision. About 2–3 percent of people develop an allergic skin reaction to LTG. This can often be prevented if the amount of LTG taken every day is increased very slowly, over several weeks, when treatment is first started. If a skin rash develops, this could be a sign of a serious allergic reaction, and it should be discussed with a doctor. Most skin rashes caused by LTG will disappear quickly if the medication is stopped or the amount taken every day is reduced.

GABAPENTIN (GBP)

Gabapentin is another relatively new drug treatment for seizures. It is contained in the brand Neurontin. GBP was originally designed to imitate the body's own substance GABA, which can suppress seizures. However, its actions on the brain are quite different from those of GABA. It seems to stop seizures by slowing the flow of calcium into nerve cells.

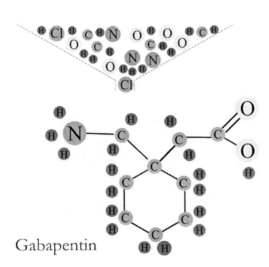

The drug is made up of:

C : Carbon

H : Hydrogen

O : Oxygen

N : Nitrogen

Gabapentin is passed out of the body by the kidneys without being broken down. It has to be replaced three times a day.

Gabapentin

Gabapentin is quickly taken up by the body and passed out again. After about 7 hours, only half the amount taken is still inside the body. Because of this, it is recommended that the drug be taken three times a day; however, it may be sufficient to take it twice a day. Gabapentin does not affect the action of other drugs (for instance, the contraceptive pill).

Gabapentin rarely causes side effects. Some people, however, develop tiredness, dizziness, or problems with balance or concentration. These side effects are usually mild and resolve after 2 weeks or so if people keep taking the tablets. Very few people have an allergic reaction to gabapentin.

OXCARBAZEPINE (OXC)

Oxcarbazepine (OXC) is chemically related to the drug carbamazepine, and it is used in a very similar way. Oxcarbazepine is contained in the brand Trileptal. Like carbamazepine, OXC may stop seizures by blocking sodium channels in the wall of nerve cells in the brain.

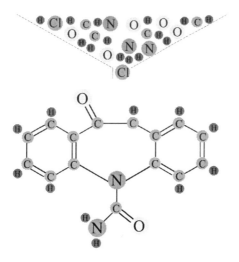

The drug is made up of:

ⓒ : Carbon
ⓗ : Hydrogen
Ⓝ : Nitrogen
o : Oxygen

Like other drugs, OXC is broken down and passed out of the body. The amount that is broken down each day has to be replaced each day.

Oxcarbazepine

Oxcarbazepine is less likely to cause side effects than carbamazepine. OXC may cause side effects in some people if they were also treated with carbamazepine. Although OXC and carbamazepine are chemically similar, they are broken down in different ways. Perhaps this is why OXC causes fewer side effects than carbamazepine. In higher doses, however, OXC can cause the same side effects as carbamazepine. Some people develop an allergic reaction to OXC. OXC weakens the effect of the contraceptive pill.

ETHOSUXIMIDE (ESM)

Ethosuximide (ESM) belongs to a group of drugs called succinimides. ESM is contained in the brand Zarontin. ESM is chemically similar to methsuximide, which is contained in the brand Celontin. Succinimides have been used for epilepsy for about 50 years. ESM is available in tablet or syrup form.

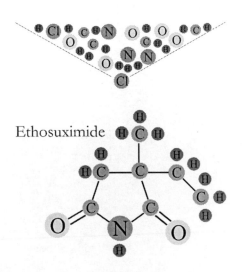

The drug is made up of:

Ⓒ : Carbon
Ⓗ : Hydrogen
Ⓞ : Oxygen
Ⓝ : Nitrogen

Ethosuximide is broken down slowly so that the whole amount needed for one day can be taken in a single dose.

Ethosuximide is mainly used for absence seizures in children and adolescents. It does not stop tonic-clonic seizures. If people also have tonic-clonic seizures, they cannot be treated with ESM alone. ESM is often combined with valproate because these two drugs work very well together.

ESM rarely causes side effects. If there are side effects, they are most likely to develop shortly after starting the drug. Very rarely, ESM may cause changes in thinking and anxiety. Like most other antiepileptic drugs, ESM can cause an allergic reaction in some people.

PRIMIDONE (PRM)

In chemical terms, primidone (PRM) is closely related to phenobarbital. The body breaks most of the PRM down to phenobarbital, so the strengths and side effects of the two drugs are very similar. PRM is contained in the brand Mysoline.

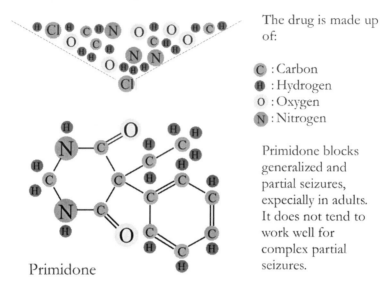

The drug is made up of:

ⓒ : Carbon
⬤ : Hydrogen
○ : Oxygen
Ⓝ : Nitrogen

Primidone blocks generalized and partial seizures, expecially in adults. It does not tend to work well for complex partial seizures.

Primidone

As with phenobarbital, the dose of primidone has to be increased and reduced slowly. The amount of PRM should not rise or fall quickly in the blood. This means that it can take weeks or months to stop PRM.

PRM has the same side effects as phenobarbital, mainly tiredness and problems with concentration. However, some people get nausea or an allergic skin reaction from PRM. Most physicians prefer phenobarbital to primidone.

LEVETIRACETAM (LEV)

Levetiracetam (LEV) is contained in the brand Keppra. LEV appears to work for many seizure types, although at the moment it is mainly used for focal seizures.

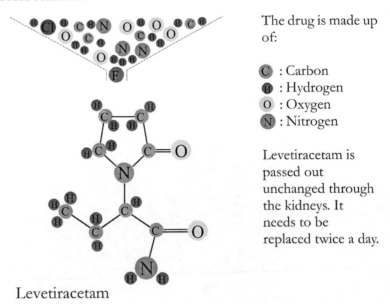

The drug is made up of:

C : Carbon
H : Hydrogen
O : Oxygen
N : Nitrogen

Levetiracetam is passed out unchanged through the kidneys. It needs to be replaced twice a day.

Levetiracetam

Little is known about how levetiracetam works in the brain. It has been shown that it does not act in the same way as any of the other antiepileptic drugs. LEV can be used on its own or in combination with other antiepileptic drugs. LEV rarely causes side effects, although some people taking it complain of tiredness, difficulty with concentration, nervousness, short temper, or difficulty with sleeping. LEV does not interfere with the action of other tablets in the body and does not change the effectiveness of the oral contraceptive pill.

PREGABALIN (PGB)

Pregabalin is a new antiepileptic drug that affects the flow of calcium into nerve cells within the brain. It makes nerve cells less able to produce epileptic discharges. The brand name is Lyrica. PGB is not bound to substances in the blood and does not seem to interact with other antiepileptic drugs. PGB is chemically related to GABA.

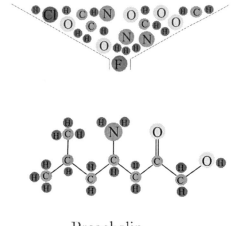

The drug is made up of:

C : Carbon
H : Hydrogen
O : Oxygen
N : Nitrogen

PGB is rapidly taken up and passed out of the body essentially unchanged through the kidneys.

Pregabalin

Tests have shown that PGB is just as effective for focal and secondary generalized seizures as other new antiepileptic drugs. It appears to be ineffective for absence seizures.

Side effects of PGB include drowsiness, tiredness, weight gain, and dizziness. Experience with the use of PGB is quite limited at present.

TIAGABINE (TGB)

Tiagabine is another relatively new drug and is contained in the brand Gabitril. It is currently only used when another antiepileptic drug (like carbamazepine) does not stop seizures on its own. It is mainly used for focal seizures in the brain.

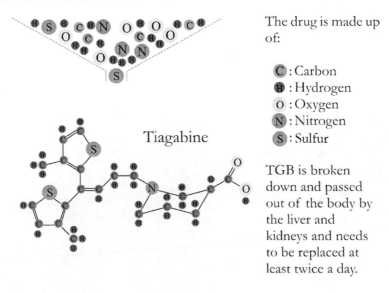

The drug is made up of:

C : Carbon
H : Hydrogen
O : Oxygen
N : Nitrogen
S : Sulfur

Tiagabine

TGB is broken down and passed out of the body by the liver and kidneys and needs to be replaced at least twice a day.

Tiagabine is quickly broken down and passed out. After 6 hours, only half the amount of TGB taken is still in the body.

Side effects are more common in people who take high doses of TGB. Most side effects come from the brain—dizziness, shakiness, and changes in thinking. Sometimes TGB also causes headaches or weakness in the legs.

Tiagabine was designed to increase the brain's own ability to block seizures. One of the main substances the body uses for this is GABA. Tiagabine is thought to act against seizures by increasing the effects of GABA in the brain. Tiagabine does not reduce the effect of the contraceptive pill.

TOPIRAMATE (TPM)

Topiramate (TPM) is a relatively new drug, which is contained in the brand Topamax. It can be used in combination with other drugs (like carbamazepine or valproate) or on its own. It is mostly used for focal seizures but it also works for primary generalized seizures.

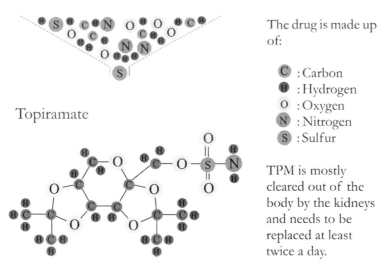

The drug is made up of:

C : Carbon
H : Hydrogen
O : Oxygen
N : Nitrogen
S : Sulfur

TPM is mostly cleared out of the body by the kidneys and needs to be replaced at least twice a day.

Topiramate

Like many other drugs, topiramate is particularly likely to cause side effects when it is first started. Most side effects come from the brain. They include tiredness, dizziness, difficulty with speaking, or problems with vision and weight loss. Sometimes people on TPM become more irritable, aggressive, or depressed than they were before. TPM can also cause tingling in the face and hands, and decreased sweating, especially in children (which can lead to elevated body temperatures). TPM increases the risk of kidney stones and glaucoma. The risk of kidney stones is smaller if people who take TPM drink plenty of fluid. Topiramate can weaken the effect of the contraceptive pill.

ACTH

ACTH is a hormone made by the body. Its full name is adrenocorti-cotropic hormone. It is contained in the brand Acthar Gel. The hormone is made naturally in the brain and is needed to help the body deal with stressful situations. It is a type of protein that cannot be taken in tablet form but has to be injected. We know quite a lot about the effects of the hormone when it is produced in response to stress. However, we do not fully understand why it stops seizures.

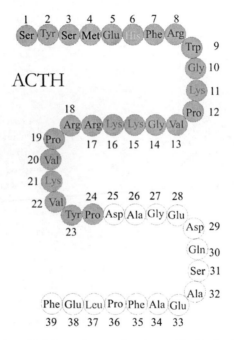

The drug is a protein, which is made up of amino acids. Each circle in the diagram stands for one amino acid. The body makes all its proteins out of about 25 different amino acids, which can be hooked together in long chains. ACTH is a small protein consisting of only 39 amino acids.

ACTH should only be used in small children with a severe type of epilepsy like West syndrome, which cannot be stopped with other drugs. It is a powerful hormone and has to be used with great care. When ACTH has to be given for several weeks, blood pressure can rise and the body is less able to fight off infections.

ACETAZOLAMIDE

Acetazolamide is a so-called "second line" antiepileptic drug that can occasionally be helpful. Acetazolamide is contained in the brands Diamox and Diamox Sequel. The drug is sometimes used when tonic-clonic seizures do not stop (status epilepticus) and when other drugs like benzodiazepines do not work. Acetazolamide is then injected into a vein. The drug is also used in several other diseases like glaucoma and periodic paralysis.

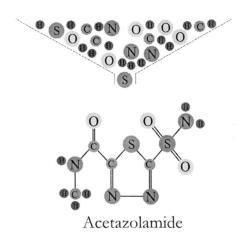

Acetazolamide

The drug is made up of:

C : Carbon
H : Hydrogen
O : Oxygen
N : Nitrogen
S : Sulfur

Acetazolamide is rapidly passed out of the body by the kidneys and has to be replaced at least three times a day.

Acetazolamide makes the kidneys pass out potassium. The way it acts against seizures is not fully understood. It causes changes in the blood and nervous tissue that are similar to those seen with the ketogenic diet (which is based on the avoidance of carbohydrates, bread, and sweets). As with the benzodiazepine group of drugs, the antiepileptic effects of acetazolamide often decrease over several months when it is taken every day. Acetazolamide often causes tingling around the mouth and in the fingers but serious side effects are rare. It belongs to the chemical group of the sulfonamides (like certain antibiotics). People with known allergic reactions against sulfonamides should avoid acetazolamide.

ZONISAMIDE (ZNS)

Zonisamide is a relatively new antiepileptic drug that can be added to drugs like carbamazepine or valproate when they do not stop seizures on their own. Zonisamide is contained in the brand Zonegran. Like many other antiepileptic drugs, it was discovered by chance. Zonisamide chemically belongs to the sulfonamides.

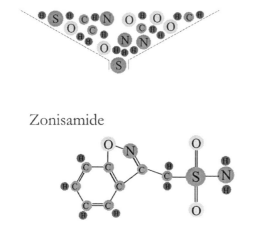

Zonisamide

The drug is made up of:

C : Carbon
H : Hydrogen
O : Oxygen
N : Nitrogen
S : Sulfur

ZNS is taken up rapidly but passed out of the body slowly. It has to be replaced several times a day.

Zonisamide can stop many types of seizures. Its mode of action is largely unknown. As with the other drugs against seizures, side effects appear more often if a greater amount of ZNS is taken every day. Typical side effects are drowsiness, tiredness, dizziness, and nervousness. Side effects usually disappear when the amount of the drug in the body is reduced. As with most other new antiepileptic drugs, it is uncertain whether the drug affects the development of babies in the womb. ZNS may also cause kidney stones, as well as reduce sweating, especially in children, leading to elevated body temperature. Like acetazolamide and certain antibiotics, Zonisamide belongs to the chemical group of sulfonamides. People who are known to be allergic to sulfonamides should not take zonisamide.

FELBAMATE (FBM)

Felbamate (FBM) is a drug against seizures that is contained in the brand Felbatol. This drug is rarely used, although it works against more seizure types than carbamazepine or phenytoin. In fact, it is not approved as a treatment for epilepsy in several countries outside the United States. In 1994, it was reported that adults taking felbamate could develop severe and possibly life-threatening blood (aplastic anemia) or liver problems. These problems were not observed in children. Treatment with FBM is sometimes considered in children with Lennox-Gastaut syndrome, a form of epilepsy that is very difficult to treat.

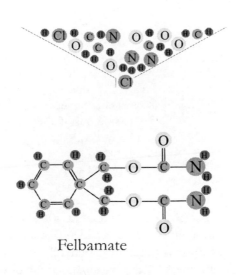

Felbamate

The drug is made up of:

C : Carbon
H : Hydrogen
O : Oxygen
N : Nitrogen

Felbamate is mainly used in children from the age of 4 and in adults when seizures have not been stopped by other drugs.

The side effects of FBM include skin rashes and changes in the blood. The skin rash can be dangerous. It sometimes occurs a few months after the tablets were first started. Small blisters in the mouth are an early sign of this skin rash. The changes in the blood are caused by the body making fewer new blood cells. FBM can also cause liver damage. Because of these possible side effects, people taking FBM have to undergo regular blood tests. FBM causes nervousness, irritability, difficulty falling asleep, and weight loss when it is taken in large doses.

VIGABATRIN (VGB)

Vigabatrin (VGB) is another antiepileptic drug that has been available for a relatively short time. It is contained in the brand Sabril, which is currently under review by the FDA. Like gabapentin, VGB was designed to imitate the body's own messenger substance GABA, which acts against seizures. The idea was to stop seizures by strengthening the effects of GABA in the brain. It is thought that VGB does this by slowing down the breakdown of GABA in the brain.

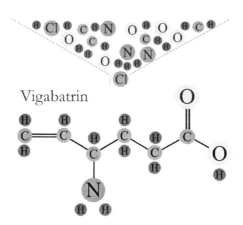

Vigabatrin

The drug is made up of:

C : Carbon
H : Hydrogen
O : Oxygen
N : Nitrogen

Vigabatrin is passed out of the body by the kidneys without being broken down. It needs to be replaced twice a day.

Vigabatrin is sometimes added on to other drugs like carbamazepine. It can be particularly effective against focal seizures that have not been stopped by other antiepileptic drugs. In spite of this advantage, it is not used very often because it damages the visual field in one out of three people. It causes vision to be restricted as if one were permanently looking through a pipe. Vision does not usually recover when VGB is stopped. In order to detect problems with vision early, people who take VGB should have their field of vision checked regularly. Other side effects include tiredness and poor concentration. Despite its side effects, vigabatrin is currently still an important treatment for a type of epilepsy called West syndrome, which affects babies and toddlers.

THIOPENTAL AND PROPOFOL (GENERAL ANESTHESIA)

There is usually no need to interrupt a seizure, because most seizures stop on their own. However, if one seizure follows on from another and status epilepticus develops, an ambulance has to be called. In most cases, status epilepticus can be stopped with benzodiazepines like lorazepam or diazepam. When these drugs do not work, phenytoin or phenobarbital is usually given next. However, these drugs also may fail to stop status. If this happens, people are given an anesthetic, as if they were having an operation.

Thiopental   Propofol

The drugs most commonly used for general anesthesia in status epilepticus to sleep are pentobarbital, thiopental, and propofol. Pentobarbital and thiopental are barbiturate drugs like phenobarbital but they are given straight into a vein. Like thiopental, propofol is usually used in the operating room for general anesthesia. Once people have been anesthetized with these drugs, normal body functions like breathing, blood pressure, and the production of urine in the kidneys have to be monitored closely. Because of this, people requiring these treatments are taken to an intensive care unit and attached to many machines. When general anesthesia is used to stop status epilepticus, people are usually kept asleep for 1 or 2 days.

THERE ARE MORE NEW ANTIEPILEPTIC DRUGS

Fosphenytoin

Fosphenytoin is a drug that can only be injected into a vein or muscles. It is contained in the brand Cerebyx. Fosphenytoin is quickly converted by the body into phenytoin. It is only used for status epilepticus or in people who cannot take phenytoin by mouth. It acts more quickly than phenytoin and causes less irritation to veins.

Lacosamide

Lacosamide (brand name Vimpat) is a new antiepileptic drug that can be added to other antiepileptic drugs if partial or secondary generalized tonic-clonic seizures continue despite treatment. It was recently approved for use in the United States for persons 17 and older. Lacosamide can stop seizures by making nerve cells electrically less excitable by acting on a particular type of sodium channel in the cell walls.

Rufinamide

Rufinamide (brand name Banzel) has recently been approved in the United States and in Europe for the treatment of patients 4 years of age and older with a particularly severe seizure disorder (Lennox-Gastaut syndrome). Rufinamide can be added to other antiepileptic drugs if they fail to control the seizures fully. The chemical structure of rufinamide is different from that of other antiepileptic drugs. It is thought that rufinamide makes nerve cells less excitable by acting on sodium channels in the cell walls.

Stiripentol

Stiripentol (brand name Diacomit) is a drug that is not yet approved by the FDA, but is approved in Europe for generalized tonic-clonic seizures in patients with severe myoclonic epilepsy in infancy (also known as Dravet's syndrome). Like clonazepam, valproate, topiramate, and phenobarbital, stiripentol appears to be effective for a range of epilepsy syndromes related to defects in a particular sodium channel gene (the SCN1A gene). Problems with the SCN1A gene often affect several members of the same family, although they may have different types of epilepsy (including isolated febrile seizures, generalized epilepsy with febriles seizures, severe myoclonic epilepsy, West syndrome, and Lennox-Gastaut syndrome).

SEIZURE MEDICINES ARE APPROVED BY THE U.S. FOOD AND DRUG ADMINISTRATION (FDA)

Not all drugs that have been proven effective for the treatment of epilepsy have also been approved by the FDA for the treatment of epilepsy. In practice, it is considered not only legal but also ethical for doctors to prescribe medicines (especially for children) that have not been FDA-approved if there is sound evidence to suggest that they are safe and effective. This so-called off-label use of seizure medicines is very common.

Many new antiepileptic drugs are being developed

New substances have to be tested. The picture shows a test protocol for a group of new substances with possible effects on epileptic seizures.

Test Protocol for New Antiepileptic Drugs

Substance	Effect	Substance	Effect	Substance	Effect	Substance	Effect
1	−	10	0	19	−	28	−
2	−	11	0	20	−	29	0
3	0	12	−	21	++	30	0
4	−	13	−	22	+	31	0
5	0	14	−	23	−	32	+
6	+	15	0	24	0	33	−
7	−	16	0	25	0	34	−
8	−	17	−	26	0	35	0
9	−	18	−	27	−	36	0

Explanation:− = brings on epileptic activity; 0 = no effect; + = weak effect on epileptic activity; ++ = strong effect on epileptic activity

Nervous tissue from a snail was treated with the new substances 1–36 to see how these substances would affect epileptic activity. The tests show that most of the substances increase epileptic activity or have no effect on it. Only substance number 21 has a strong action against epileptic activity. Further tests have to be performed to check that this substance is not poisonous, for instance to the heart or for a baby in the womb. Substance number 21 can only be given to humans once it has proven safe in many further tests.

3.4 SIDE EFFECTS

DRUGS SHOULD STOP SEIZURES; ALL OTHER EFFECTS ARE SIDE EFFECTS

Many antiepileptic drugs slow people down in their thinking or make them feel tired. Antiepileptic drugs are not given to make people feel less anxious or make them sleepy, so these effects are side effects.

There are risks with everything we do.

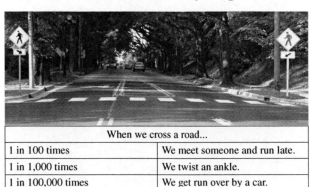

When we cross a road...	
1 in 100 times	We meet someone and run late.
1 in 1,000 times	We twist an ankle.
1 in 100,000 times	We get run over by a car.

Some antiepileptic drugs cause tiredness or drowsiness more often than others. Whereas these problems are rarely caused by lamotrigine, valproate, carbamazepine, or phenytoin, they are common with phenobarbital or primidone. The first question in the process of choosing an antiepileptic drug for a particular person is which drugs would be more likely to stop the seizures. However, other issues are important too—such as which side effects could develop and what impact they could have on someone's life. Older adults, for instance, may cope better with tiredness than a child going to school. In a woman who might want to have a baby, it is best to choose a drug that would be safe to take during pregnancy. People who need to take tablets for other medical problems may not be able to take certain antiepileptic drugs.

SIDE EFFECTS ARE MOSTLY A NUISANCE BUT CAN ALSO BE DANGEROUS

A particularly nasty and unpleasant side effect may turn out to be relatively harmless, whereas a side effect that was hardly noticeable, and did not seem especially troublesome at first, could turn out to be dangerous. How ill someone feels with a side effect does not always show how dangerous it is. It is best to discuss side effects with a doctor.

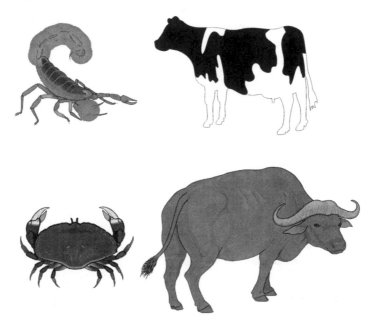

It is often not easy to say how serious a side effect is based on its first appearance. The same is true of animals. Scorpions look similar to crabs; cows look similar to wild buffaloes. While crabs and cows are fairly harmless, scorpions can be poisonous and wild buffaloes are so dangerous that even lions keep their distance from them.

TREATMENT SHOULD PREVENT SEIZURES WITHOUT CAUSING SIDE EFFECTS

Many people who go to see a doctor about seizures are worried that antiepileptic drugs are tranquilizers or sedatives given to calm them down. They are often concerned that they could get addicted to them. Some people think that drugs cannot really help with seizures unless they also cause unpleasant side effects. However, none of this is true.

Reading the drug information sheet prepared by the FDA, called the "package insert," may provide reassurance to some. Information sheets may cause some people to worry even more about side effects.

Drug information sheets contain lists of side effects. Drug manufacturers must, by law, inform users about any possible side effects, even if they are rare. This makes it difficult for people who have to take the drugs to judge the actual risk of getting side effects.

brand name   pharmaceutical
name of the drug   company

Information for Patients

What you need to know about the drug

What is in your medicine?

Who makes your medicine?

What this medicine is used for

Before taking your medicine ask yourself the following questions:

Are you taking any of the following?

Medication users may be as uncertain about the effects or side effects of their tablets as people who try to read this drug information sheet, which was blurred deliberately to illustrate how unclear the included information can be.

SIDE EFFECTS ARE GENERALLY UNWANTED EFFECTS

All drugs can cause side effects but it is impossible to know who will get them. Some side effects are more troublesome than others.

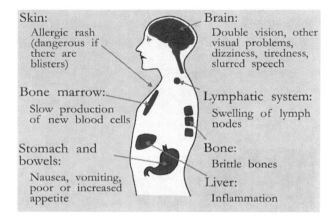

Skin:
Allergic rash (dangerous if there are blisters)

Brain:
Double vision, other visual problems, dizziness, tiredness, slurred speech

Bone marrow:
Slow production of new blood cells

Lymphatic system:
Swelling of lymph nodes

Stomach and bowels:
Nausea, vomiting, poor or increased appetite

Bone:
Brittle bones

Liver:
Inflammation

Drugs are taken up by the blood and delivered to all the parts of the body, not just the brain. For the most part, the other organs are not affected by antiepileptic drugs. Sometimes, however, antiepileptic drugs cause reactions like those described in the picture.

Many drug reactions resolve with time and are so mild that treatment does not have to be changed. Other reactions may be troublesome but less risky or unpleasant than seizures, so that people put up with them. However, there are some drug reactions that are dangerous or that interfere too much with daily life. In such cases, the drug usually has to be stopped, or people have to take a smaller dose.

Side effects should be discussed with a doctor.

ANTIEPILEPTIC DRUGS CAN CAUSE SEIZURES

Antiepileptic drugs can sometimes cause seizures because each substance acts on the brain in a number of different ways. The main effect will make seizures less likely but other effects may make seizures worse. Usually, the protection against seizures cancels out any effects that could actually cause seizures. The picture shows that, during weeks 1–4, the antiepileptic drug stops seizures more strongly than it makes them happen. If the two effects are added up, the drug is beneficial because it reduces the overall number of seizures the person has.

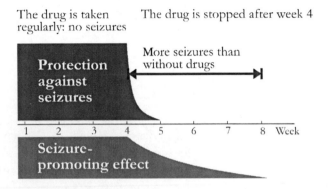

In this example, the antiepileptic drug is stopped suddenly after 4 weeks. The protection against seizures disappears more quickly than the effects of the drug that may cause seizures. In the 5th and 6th weeks only the seizure-promoting effect is left, so it is likely that more seizures will occur than if no drug had been taken. Stopping antiepileptic drugs suddenly can cause status epilepticus. This is a very dangerous condition in which one seizure is followed by another before the person has fully recovered.

THE DOSE OF ANTIEPILEPTIC DRUGS SHOULD ONLY BE LOWERED SLOWLY

The dose of an antiepileptic drug may have to be lowered because of side effects. If these are severe, and a drug has to be stopped suddenly, seizures can be prevented by taking another drug which works quickly. However, the risk of an increase of seizures or of status epilepticus is much lower if drugs can be reduced slowly. If possible, antiepileptic drugs should therefore always be tapered off and never stopped suddenly.

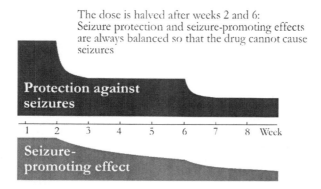

The dose is halved after weeks 2 and 6:
Seizure protection and seizure-promoting effects are always balanced so that the drug cannot cause seizures

Protection against seizures

1   2   3   4   5   6   7   8   Week

Seizure-promoting effect

The diagram shows that the overall effect of antiepileptic drugs is to stop seizures if the dose is reduced slowly (in the example, the total dose is halved two times). Antiepileptic drugs should be stopped slowly because stopping them suddenly can cause seizures. They should be started slowly because starting them quickly can cause side effects.

> If antiepileptic drugs are taken regularly as they are prescribed, they only cause seizures only very rarely.

THE DOSE OF ANTIEPILEPTIC DRUGS SHOULD ONLY BE INCREASED SLOWLY

Treatment with antiepileptic drugs is intended to stop seizures completely without causing side effects.

Side effects are more likely with higher doses of medication. For this reason, it is important to find the lowest dose of medication that is necessary to stop seizures. The best way of finding this dose is to increase treatment slowly until seizures stop. A seizure diary can help in these problems.

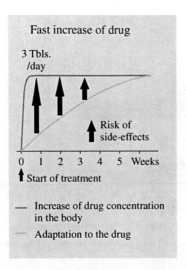 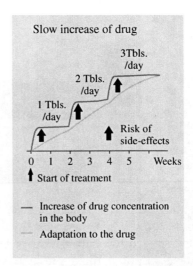

Drugs are taken up by the blood and carried to all organs of the body. The organs get used to or "adapt" to the drug. This adaptation takes place without causing problems in most cases, although this process takes time. The risk of side effects can be reduced if medication is increased slowly, so the body can adjust to it.

As an analogy, this is similar to how the body reacts to very cold water. It could be dangerous as well as very unpleasant to jump into a cold mountain lake on a hot day. It is safer to cool the body more slowly.

ANTIEPILEPTIC DRUGS CAN CHANGE THE EFFECTS OF OTHER MEDICATIONS

Antiepileptic drugs can weaken or strengthen the effects of other tablets. The oral contraceptive pill, for instance, contains hormones that ensure that women cannot become pregnant. These hormones (like many drugs against seizures) are broken down and passed out of the body by the liver.

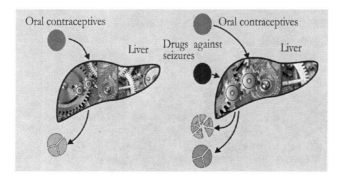

If women take oral contraceptives and antiepileptic drugs, the antiepileptic drugs can cause the machinery in the liver to work more quickly. The body uses this machinery to break down drugs, including oral contraceptives and antiepileptic drugs. This means that oral contraceptives are broken down and passed out of the body more quickly. They are therefore less effective, and the risk of becoming pregnant increases. Women who wish to take oral contraceptives together with antiepileptic drugs either have to take a higher dose of hormones to stop pregnancy, use a barrier method of contraception, or switch to a type of antiepileptic drug that does not make the liver work more quickly. They should discuss this with their doctor.

> **Antiepileptic drugs can reduce the effect of the oral contraceptive pill.**

ANTIEPILEPTIC DRUGS CAN CHANGE THE EFFECTS OF ALCOHOL

There is a complicated relationship between alcohol, epileptic seizures, and antiepileptic drugs. Most people with epilepsy may drink one or two glasses of beer or wine without any bad effects. However, it is dangerous for them to drink a large amount of alcohol. This can cause an increase in seizures. People who are addicted to alcohol may be at particular risk of this because drinking alcohol can make it harder for them to remember to take their antiepileptic drugs regularly.

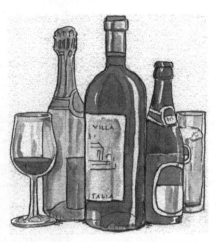

Alcohol addiction also puts people at risk of alcohol withdrawal seizures and status epilepticus. Anyone who has to take antiepileptic drugs and wants to drink alcohol has to remember that alcohol increases side effects, so that they may feel drunk very quickly.

Antiepileptic drugs can also increase the effects of other drugs. This may be helpful when a combination of antiepileptic drugs is used to treat people with particularly difficult-to-control seizures. However, it may also be an unwanted effect, for instance, where antiepileptic drugs increase the effects of tablets for heart conditions. Other tablets can also increase the effects or side effects of antiepileptic drugs. Because of this, before new medication is started, it is important to tell doctors about all current drug treatments as well as about over-the-counter medications, herbs, and dietary supplements that may be used.

It is best only to take drugs that are really necessary.

OTHER MEDICATION CAN CHANGE THE EFFECTS OF ANTIEPILEPTIC DRUGS

People with epilepsy may have other conditions that need to be treated with medication. When using other medication, they need to consider the effect this can have on their epilepsy and antiepileptic drugs. A number of drugs can make epilepsy worse. These include medication for asthma (theophylline, aminophylline), antibiotics (lindane, penicillin), local anesthetics when injected into blood vessels (lidocaine, procaine), certain drugs for depression (bupropion), and many others.

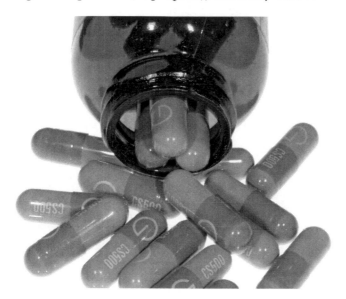

With permission from Nick Atkins

People with epilepsy who suddenly experience a worsening of their seizures should ask themselves whether they have taken any additional medication—including herbal medication or dietary supplements (such as St. John's wort).

Some medications reduce the seizure threshold in the brain. Others cause the liver or kidneys to pass antiepileptic drugs out of the body more quickly, so that the dose of antiepileptic drugs has to be increased.

HERBS AND DIETARY SUPPLEMENTS CAN CHANGE THE EFFECTS OF ANTIEPILEPTIC DRUGS

In past centuries, various herbs were used as remedies and many of the drugs we use today are based on herbal remedies (for instance, aspirin). When herbal remedies are used today, they are rarely as effective as the prescribed medicines. Some common herbs appear to increase seizure activity. Essential oils distilled from common plants are widely used in aromatherapy and massage oils. Though "natural," they are not harmless. For example, essential oils made from eucalyptus, fennel, hyssop, pennyroyal, rosemary, sage, savin, tansy, thuja, turpentine, and wormwood may cause seizures. People with epilepsy should avoid the essential oils of these herbs and products.

IF THERE ARE SIDE EFFECTS, TREATMENT SHOULD BE CHECKED

Are the side effects dangerous?

Side effects are only rarely so dangerous that treatment has to be stopped immediately; however, this determination should be made by the physician. In such cases, people may have to stay in the hospital because there can be more seizures or even status epilepticus.

Would the side effects resolve with time if the treatment was continued?

Some people are particularly sensitive to certain drugs, but their body may get used to them. However, people may also be allergic to drugs. Most allergic reactions show up as a skin rash, which may be itchy. When drug allergies are dangerous they usually affect the inside of the mouth and can cause blisters on the skin. People who experience this should contact their doctor right away.

Is the dose too high?

Many side effects go away if the dose of the tablets can be reduced. The level at which side effects occur for any given person cannot be predicted. "Dose-related" side effects include dizziness, tiredness, and poor vision. That means that it is likely the side effects would worsen if the dose was increased and improve if the dose was reduced. People may also feel that their thinking is slow. In high doses, most antiepileptic drugs can cause nausea and vomiting.

3.5 OTHER TREATMENTS THAT MAY HELP

EPILEPSY CAN BE TREATED WITH ELECTRICAL STIMULATION OF THE "VAGUS NERVE"

To do this, an electrical stimulator (which works like a pacemaker for the heart) is inserted under the skin in the left upper chest. The machine is linked by a wire under the skin to the "vagus nerve" in the neck. This nerve normally carries information from the brain to the organs in the chest and stomach and information from the same organs to the brain. The electrical impulses from the stimulator are carried into the brain. These impulses affect the nerve cells of the brain, so that there may be fewer seizures.

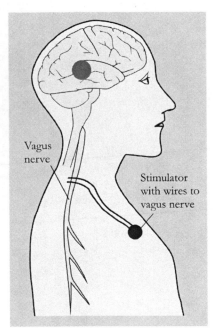

Vagus nerve

Stimulator with wires to vagus nerve

Worldwide, vagus nerve stimulators have been implanted in over 50,000 people. About one-third of them have benefited from the stimulator and have had fewer seizures. In another third, seizures may lessen in intensity.

Some people also feel better about themselves with a stimulator in place. It can take up to 1 year until the full effect of vagus nerve stimulation is seen.

> **Vagus nerve stimulation can reduce the number of seizures but rarely stops them.**

RADIATION CAN BE USED TO TREAT AN EPILEPTIC FOCUS

The gamma knife is a medical instrument that simultaneously sends out over 200 beams of radiation. The beams enter the brain from different directions, but they are focused on one small target area in the center. Each individual beam is weak but the radiation is strong where all the beams meet in the brain. It is not clear what exactly happens to nerve cells that have been hit by the full force of the radiation. It seems that their metabolism changes.

Just like conventional surgery, gamma knife treatment for epilepsy is considered only after carefully weighing the advantages and disadvantages for each individual person. The target for radiation is usually identified using magnetic resonance imaging (MRI).

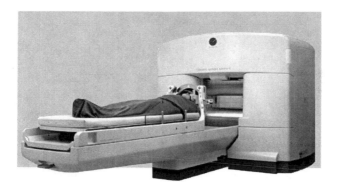

Treatment usually consists of a single session of radiation and takes only around half an hour. After this, people are observed in the hospital because they can develop swelling of the brain (edema), which may need to be treated with drugs. One or two weeks later, people can return to their usual daily activities. Gamma knife treatment seems to be particularly useful when epileptic seizures are caused by abnormal blood vessels. However, experience with the use of the gamma knife is still limited. Gamma knife treatment does not stop seizures immediately. When treatment has been effective, seizures stop after 1–3 years.

IF SEIZURE TRIGGERS CAN BE FOUND, THEY CAN SOMETIMES BE AVOIDED

Sometimes, just taking antiepileptic drugs regularly is not enough. It can be worthwhile to try to work out whether there are particular circumstances that make seizures more likely. Many people who have epilepsy know of situations or feelings that can bring on seizures. It is well recognized that flickering light, lack of sleep, drinking too much alcohol, or certain moods can help to start seizures for many people with epilepsy. However, the particular situations in which seizures occur can vary from one person to another.

Often people feel depressed, drained, or unusually tired before one of their seizures.

January				February				March			
6	12	18	hours	6	12	18	hours	6	12	18	hours

(A seizure diary grid with days 1–31 listed in each month column.)

Some triggering factors do not always lead to seizures and are therefore harder to spot. A seizure diary can help to find out about situations in which seizures are particularly likely to happen. Sometimes such situations can be avoided, so that seizures are prevented. If this works well and over a long period of time, it may even be possible to reduce or stop antiepileptic drugs. On the other hand, people should not stop doing everything they enjoy out of fear that it may cause a seizure. Some people may prefer higher doses of antiepileptic drugs, so that they can continue to do the things they enjoy doing, as long as they go about these activities with common sense.

SOME PEOPLE CAN LEARN TO INFLUENCE THE ACTIVITY OF THEIR NERVE CELLS

During a seizure warning or aura, epileptic activity spreads from the damaged nerve cells, which first start the seizure, to nerve cells that are otherwise healthy. It is sometimes possible to keep these healthy cells busy with something else, so that they cannot become involved in the seizure. This can be done by concentrating on particular images, music, or words. People may try to clench their fist if seizures start there with a tingling sensation. Often people work out how they can stop seizures without any help from others. If a method for stopping seizures has been found, it is important to train the brain by using it every time a seizure warning is felt. This takes a lot of effort and patience.

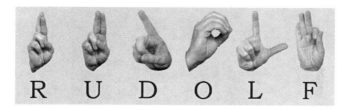

Often, people have to try many different ways of stopping seizures until they find one that works. The person in the picture has learned to stop seizures by concentrating on spelling the name "Rudolf" or other words in sign language whenever he feels a seizure coming on. This has reduced the number of seizures quite a lot.

Unfortunately, such methods of stopping seizures work only in very few people. They can work only if there is enough time between the first warning (aura) and the start of the seizure.

> Suppressing seizures is hard work, but it can help people who have epileptic seizures with auras.

THE EEG CAN HELP PEOPLE LEARN HOW TO STOP SEIZURES

The EEG, which shows the electric activity of the brain, can be used to teach some people to suppress their seizures using "biofeedback." In this process, a person looks at the monitor of a computer while the EEG is being recorded from his brain and fed into the computer. The computer is programmed to change the picture on the monitor when a certain type of signal is present in the EEG. The person is encouraged to change the picture. In this way, he learns to produce the desired EEG signal. People are then encouraged to produce this particular type of EEG activity on a daily basis.

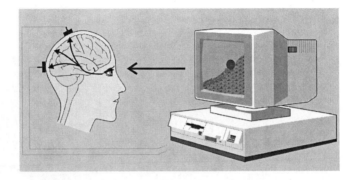

Unfortunately, only very few people with epilepsy can stop their seizures using the biofeedback method. Some people cannot learn how to influence their EEG activity. In other people, the method has no apparent effect on seizures.

Some people can stop their seizures by learning the biofeedback method and producing the right EEG signal.

PSYCHOLOGICAL TREATMENT CAN HELP SOME PEOPLE WITH EPILEPSY

Seizures sometimes happen when people are very excited or stressed. They may be able to avoid such excitement and stress. This may require help from a psychologist or psychotherapist. For instance, if someone is afraid of open spaces, which they cannot always avoid, it is possible to reduce anxiety by desensitization. Desensitization may be based on the gradual introduction of open spaces that were avoided before. Sometimes seizures disappear together with the person's previous fears.

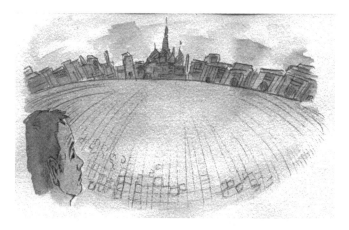

Occasionally, seizures are caused by overbreathing related to anxiety or excitement. Overbreathing leads to a reduction in the carbon dioxide level in the blood. Low carbon dioxide can cause seizures in some persons. People can learn to control their breathing so that they do not put themselves at risk of a seizure. They may also be told to breathe back air from a paper bag placed over their mouth. This increases the amount of carbon dioxide in the blood back to normal levels.

DIETS CAN LOWER THE FREQUENCY OF EPILEPTIC SEIZURES

A "ketogenic diet" causes changes in the body's metabolism that make seizures less likely. It is not known exactly how this diet works. It consists of fat and protein and is similar to the Atkins diet, which some people use to lose weight. Sugar has to be avoided. Cheese, meat, butter, eggs, and oil are good. Bread, cake, sweets, fruit, and certain vegetables have to be reduced or stopped by people trying to follow the rules of the ketogenic diet.

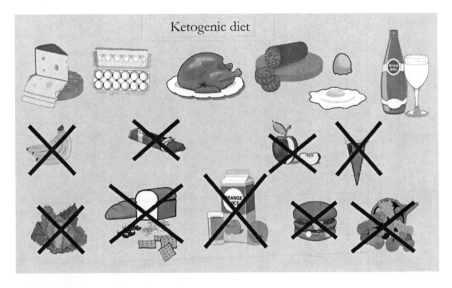

This diet is not a "fad" or "quack" diet, but rather an alternative or additional medical treatment that has been proven to work in some people with epilepsy when antiepileptic drugs have not been effective. Its effects start after a few days. The evidence that this diet works for epilepsy is strongest for children. Little is known about the long-term effects of the diet. Other diets or diet supplements are sometimes advised for people with epilepsy, but none have ever been proven to work and some very strict diets can be harmful.

SOMETIMES CERTAIN SMELLS AND TASTES CAN STOP SEIZURES

Some people try to find a smell or taste to block the cells that produce epileptic activity in the brain. When they have an aura, they either sniff the scent from a small bottle or they imagine smelling a particular smell. It is important that people take a careful look at whether this approach actually reduces the number of their seizures. They can use their seizure diary for this. Seizures can also be made worse by certain smells.

Example

Mrs. S. has had secondary generalized tonic-clonic seizures for 26 years. Antiepileptic drugs have not controlled her seizures. The seizures always start with warning symptoms. At first, Mrs. S. feels confused in a particular way, and then she becomes aware of a foul smell that other people cannot smell. Mrs. S.'s doctor tells her about people who were able to train their brain to control seizures by using a particular scent. Mrs. S. decides to open and sniff a bottle of lavender oil every time she has a seizure warning. After persisting for several weeks, her seizures stop when she uses her bottle. Some months later, she does not have her bottle on hand when she has a seizure warning. Instead of experiencing the usual foul smell, she only smells lavender and there is no tonic-clonic seizure. She stops using the scent bottle and continues to have attacks, where she immediately smells lavender and after which there are no other seizures. Eventually, she stops smelling lavender as well. Her brain has learned to stop her seizures.

The same smell may stop seizures in one person and cause them in another. Often people can predict whether a particular smell will make their seizures better or worse. Sometimes it is also possible to try to influence seizures through other senses (seeing, hearing, touching).

ACUPUNCTURE HAS NOT PROVEN SUCCESSFUL AT PREVENTING SEIZURES

It is not fully understood how acupuncture needles stimulate or calm down the nervous system. Electro-acupuncture uses electricity to stimulate a particular part of the skin. It is easy to imagine that this can stimulate nerve fibers, which could have an effect on epileptic activity.

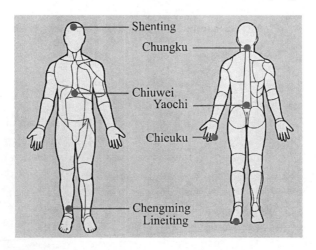

Studies of the effects of acupuncture have not produced clear results. In one study, a group of people with epilepsy was treated by Chinese acupuncture specialists. Only one-half of the group was treated with true acupuncture. Stimulation of the true acupuncture points led to an over 50 percent reduction of seizures in 39 percent of the people treated. However 33 percent of the patients treated with true acupuncture had an increase of over 50 percent in their epileptic seizures.

3.6 EPILEPSY SURGERY

DURING EPILEPSY SURGERY, A PART OF THE BRAIN IS REMOVED

Epilepsy surgery is done only in specialized centers. Operations are never without risk. Because of this, people can only have an operation for epilepsy if a number of conditions are met.

Epilepsy surgery can be considered if . . .

- Seizures are so severe that they badly affect a person's quality of life.
- The seizures arise from a part of the brain that is amenable to surgical treatment.
- A number of antiepileptic drugs have been tried but seizures have continued.
- Seizures can only be stopped by using antiepileptic drugs in doses that cause troublesome side effects.

It is never easy to decide whether to go ahead with epilepsy surgery. People considering surgery always have to go through a lot of tests. Some of these tests have their own risks.

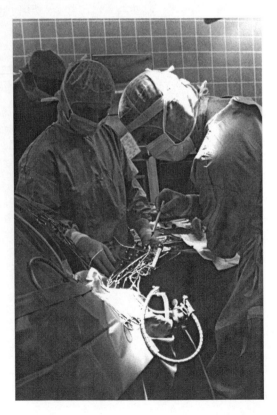

WHERE DO SEIZURES START IN THE BRAIN?

Sometimes, the seizure symptoms suggest where seizures start in the brain. If seizures always start with flashes of light, for instance, it is likely that the epileptic activity begins and spreads from the vision center of the brain. If seizures begin with a sudden memory from the past, they are likely to come from the memory centers of the brain in the temporal lobes.

THE EEG CAN HELP TO FIND THE SOURCE OF SEIZURES

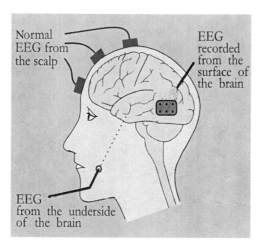

To find out which part of the brain epileptic activity comes from, seizures have to be observed with an EEG. This means that people may have to be attached to an EEG machine as long as it takes to record several typical seizures. To make seizures more likely during such a recording, antiepileptic drugs may be tapered or stopped in the hospital.

In some cases, the EEG has to be recorded straight from the surface of the brain rather than the scalp. To do this, holes have to be drilled into the head and wires are pushed onto the surface of the brain. Sometimes the EEG is also recorded from the underside of the brain using wires inserted through the cheeks. Recording the EEG from the surface of the brain involves an operation that has risks.

It is important to be certain exactly where seizures start in the brain when epilepsy surgery is being considered.

MRI IMAGES CAN SHOW WHERE SEIZURES START

Often MRI (magnetic resonance imaging) images provide some clue about the source of seizures within the brain. The MRI may, for instance, show changes of the shape or structure of one particular part of the brain. If such changes are seen in an area of the brain in which there are also abnormalities in the EEG, it is likely that seizures come from this part of the brain.

EPILEPSY SURGERY MUST NOT DISTURB THE NORMAL WORKING OF THE BRAIN

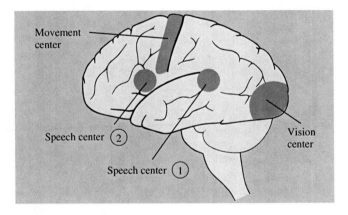

In this picture, the movement, speech, and vision centers of the brain are marked.

Surgery in these centers would damage one of the important functions of the brain. If, for instance, the speech center (1) was damaged during an operation, there would be problems with understanding the meaning of language. The person affected would hear people talking to him, but he would not understand and he would be unable to answer back. This would be very disabling. Therefore, one could not consider epilepsy surgery if the place where seizures came from was very close to this speech center.

Some functions are performed by both halves of the brain, so healthy parts of the brain can take over after an operation. Sometimes it is possible to check whether a certain part of the brain is needed for an important function during an operation. This can be done by stimulating the surface of the brain with a low electrical current.

TESTING FUNCTIONS OF THE BRAIN CAN ALSO HELP TO SHOW WHERE SEIZURES START IN THE BRAIN

Certain parts of the left temporal lobe are important for remembering words. When this area is damaged, the memory for words can work less well. Since seizures start from a damaged area in the brain, problems with word memory can point to the left temporal lobe as the area where seizures start.

By testing brain functions, neuropsychologists can possibly spot an area which works less well than expected. There are memory tests for words, images or faces, tests for the ability to copy and describe images or to carry out complicated tasks or movements, and tests of the reaction to commands.

Memory Test for Words

Word list read out	Hit, Side, Bark, Shade, Gauge, Pause, Start, Stuff, Mile, Fall
Words learned initially	Hit, Shade, Pause, Start, Fall
Words remembered after 30 minutes	Hit, Pause, Start, Fall

The diagram shows the result of a word memory test. The word list at the top was read aloud several times by the examiner. Immediately afterwards, the person undergoing the test had learned only five of the words. Half an hour later, when he was asked to recall the words again, he could still remember only four words.

During the test in the diagram, most people learn nine or ten of the words. The poor result of the person in this test shows that there is damage in the part of the brain that deals with memory. The fact that the person tested found it difficult to learn words, but remembered them well later, suggests that the damage is in the outer layer of the left temporal lobe and not in the hippocampus.

THE WADA TEST CAN PREVENT DAMAGE TO THE SPEECH CENTERS OF THE BRAIN

The Wada test (or "intracarotid amobarbital test") is a way of finding out which parts of the brain are important for speech and memory. It is named after Juhn A. Wada, a Japanese epileptologist. The test consists of two steps. First, the artery, which supplies the area of the brain to be examined, is inspected by angiography. This is a procedure in which a thin plastic line is placed into an artery in the groin and then moved up slowly to the arteries that lead to the brain. Dye, which can be seen on an X-ray machine, is injected to show the artery.

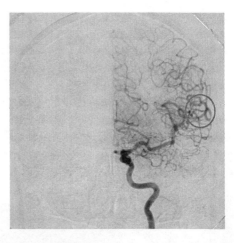

The circle in the picture marks the region which would have to be removed by epilepsy surgery. However, it could contain the speech center of the brain.

In the second step of the Wada test, the drug amobarbital is injected into the artery. The drug blocks for a short time all nerve cells supplied with blood by that artery. If speech is produced by the area marked in the picture, the person will be unable to speak after the drug injection. This means that surgery on this part of the brain would likely also damage speech.

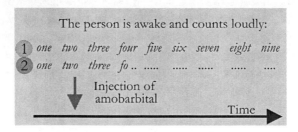

The person is awake and counts loudly:

1. one two three four five six seven eight nine
2. one two three fo.. ....

   ↓ Injection of amobarbital

   Time →

Two people are counting. In case (1) amobarbital has no effect. In case (2) speech comes from the marked area in picture.

THERE IS NO GUARANTEE THAT SURGERY WILL STOP SEIZURES

People who want to have epilepsy surgery have to undergo a lot of tests to ensure that they are likely to benefit from an operation. However, even if the tests go well, there is no guarantee that the seizures will stop. Whether seizures stop will only become clear after the operation. It takes several months before one can be confident that surgery has worked and the seizures have stopped. Of all people who have epilepsy surgery, only 60 percent become completely free of seizures. Sometimes it is not possible to cut out the whole epileptic area; sometimes the true source of epileptic seizures in the brain is missed during the operation.

Example

When he was 6 months old, Mr. J. had a seizure while he was ill with a high temperature. Until he was 3 years old, he had further seizures when he had fever. When he was 15, he developed attacks that began with an unpleasant sensation in his stomach. Sometimes he would go blank for a minute or two. At 18, he had such an attack but it was followed by a tonic-clonic seizure. Despite taking antiepileptic drugs, he continued to have three seizures every week. Mr. J. was evaluated for epilepsy surgery. EEG recordings over several days showed that seizures probably started in the left temporal lobe. On MRI pictures, the left temporal lobe looked smaller than the right. To be sure of the source of the seizures, electrodes were placed on the surface of the brain. This showed that seizures came from a part of the brain that was far enough away from the speech center to consider an operation. During surgery, a part of the left temporal lobe was removed. Mr. J. became free of seizures. However, he still has to take antiepileptic drugs.

Whether people benefit from epilepsy surgery depends on the type and cause of seizures, and where seizures come from in the brain.

EPILEPSY SURGERY IS COMMONLY PERFORMED ON THE TEMPORAL LOBES

Seizures that do not stop with antiepileptic drugs often start in the temporal lobes. Compared to other parts of the brain, the temporal lobes are relatively easy to study with tests. This means that it is less difficult to evaluate people with temporal lobe epilepsy for epilepsy surgery.

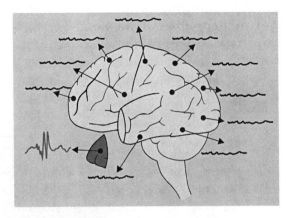

The picture shows that epileptic EEG signals come from the tip of the temporal lobe (also known as the "temporal pole"). Everywhere else, the EEG is normal.

The part of the brain that will be taken out at epilepsy surgery is shown. In most operations on the temporal lobe, the hippocampus is removed because seizures often come from there. In some people, seizures stop only if the hippocampus is taken out.

EPILEPTIC ACTIVITY CAN BE CAUSED BY ALL KINDS OF CHANGES IN THE BRAIN

The list of changes in the brain that can cause epilepsy is long. It includes scars, brain tumors, and poorly formed brain tissue or blood vessels. If these abnormalities can be taken out, seizures often stop. Sometimes surgery is not just performed to stop seizures but to remove dangerous causes (like tumors or weak blood vessels). In such cases the changes can often be seen so clearly on scans or even with the naked eye during an operation that fewer tests than usual may be necessary before surgery.

EPILEPSY SURGERY IN CHILDREN OFTEN INVOLVES TAKING OUT POORLY FORMED PARTS OF THE BRAIN

Some children develop seizures that affect one-half of the body. These seizures are often difficult to treat with antiepileptic drugs. The seizures are caused by severe changes in the opposite half of the brain. The changes may have been caused by poor development of the brain or by inflammation. In many cases, the arm and leg on the side of the body involved in the seizures are stiff, weak, or clumsy between seizures.

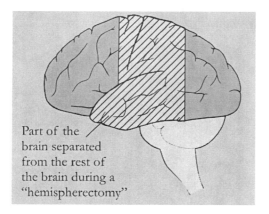

Part of the brain separated from the rest of the brain during a "hemispherectomy"

The striped area in the picture shows the part of the brain that is removed or separated from the rest of the brain during a "hemispherectomy."

In most cases, it is not known what caused the poor development or the inflammation of a part of the brain. However, it is clear that the damaged parts of the brain can stop the healthy parts of the brain from working normally. Children with severe changes in one half of their brain often do not develop well. They may even lose skills they had before they developed epilepsy. If a "hemispherectomy" can be performed, 80 percent of these children become free of seizures. They may also become more certain in their movements and able to learn much better. The improvement is often very remarkable. Children can recover lost skills much better than adults.

> Surgery works best in children who are younger and who have not had seizures for long.

A CALLOSOTOMY INVOLVES CUTTING SOME OF THE NERVE FIBERS WITHIN THE BRAIN

Rarely, an epileptic area in one half of the brain can irritate a second area in the opposite half of the brain. Epileptic activity can then spread from there to the rest of the brain. The picture shows how epileptic activity first spreads from A to B and then to the whole brain. Seizures spreading in this way can sometimes be improved by cutting the nerve fibers connecting A and B. However, such operations rarely stop seizures altogether. Sometimes seizures decrease at first but then return over the months and years following surgery.

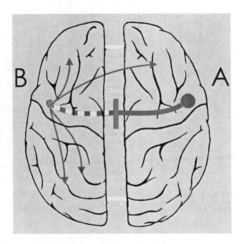

During a callosotomy, some of the nerve fibers connecting the left and the right halves of the brain are cut. The place where this cut is made is marked. Once the cut has been made, the epileptic area in the right half of the brain cannot stimulate the area in the left half. This stops the seizure from becoming generalized.

Example

Mr. G. underwent a callosotomy 50 years ago, when epilepsy surgery first started. At this time, the nerve fibers connecting the right half of the brain with the left were sometimes cut completely. The operation improved Mr. G.'s seizures, but afterwards, the left half of Mr. G.'s brain did not always "know" what the right half was up to. With his eyes closed, for instance, he was unable to name things that he was holding in his left hand (because feeling with the left hand is dealt with in the right half of the brain whereas naming things is dealt with in the left half).

EPILEPSY SURGERY IS USUALLY OFFERED WHEN THERE IS A GOOD CHANCE OF STOPPING SEIZURES

Operations are most successful when seizures come from changes in the brain that can be seen on brain images, and that can be removed completely. The removal of abnormal brain cells does not cause problems with the normal working of the brain. Since epileptic tissue can disturb the normal brain cells around it, epilepsy surgery may even improve brain function.

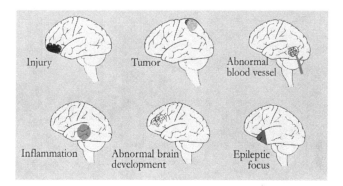

One of the drawbacks of epilepsy surgery is that once a part of the brain has been removed, it cannot be put back. In most operations, some healthy brain tissue is removed together with the epileptic area. Sometimes this causes problems with the normal working of the brain. The risk of losing functions like memory or speech can be reduced by tests, but it cannot be completely abolished. Also, there may be surgical complications, such as unexpected bleeding or infection. Lastly, the epileptic focus may not be removed completely during the operation, so that seizures may continue after surgery.

A decision about epilepsy surgery is based on many factors.

INTERRUPTION OF NERVE FIBERS BY SUBPIAL TRANSSECTIONS

The "pia mater" is the soft inner layer of the lining of the brain. Sometimes epilepsy surgery involves making small cuts ("transsections") in the surface of the brain, just underneath the pia mater ("subpial"). Such transsections are performed when the area of brain where seizures start cannot be taken out completely. For instance, if epileptic activity started in the speech areas of the brain, the production or understanding of speech would be damaged if the epileptic focus was removed.

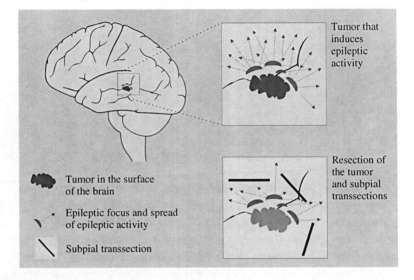

Tumor that induces epileptic activity

Resection of the tumor and subpial transsections

Tumor in the surface of the brain

Epileptic focus and spread of epileptic activity

Subpial transsection

Transsections can help the brain to block epileptic seizures because epileptic activity spreads through nerve fibers that run along the surface of the brain. Important brain functions like speech or movement, however, rely mainly on nerve fibers that connect the surface with the central parts of the brain. In many ways, the surface of the brain (the cortex) acts like a screen on which a picture of the world is projected from the inside. Small cuts in the screen would not interfere much with the projected picture.

4

EPILEPSY IN EVERYDAY LIFE

4.1 RISK AND PREJUDICE

PEOPLE WITH EPILEPSY CAN FACE PREJUDICE

Centuries ago, people with epilepsy were thought to be possessed by demons. The picture shows how the devil is being exorcised from a woman with epilepsy. The devil is flying away from the woman.

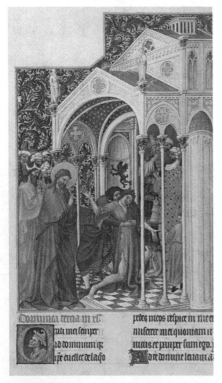

The miniature (Folio 166 recto) from the book of hours, "Les Trés Riches Heures" of Johann von Frankreich (Duc de Berry, 1340–1416).

Even today there are things that are said and thought about people with epilepsy that are wrong and can make life difficult for those who have to live with seizures.

The following statements about epilepsy are true.

- People with epilepsy have the same range of intelligence as people without epilepsy.
- Epilepsy does not cause aggression.
- Epilepsy is not a mental illness.
- Most types of epilepsy are not inherited.

The prejudice people with epilepsy face reflects not only how little the general public knows about epilepsy, but also the insecurity and anxiety many people feel when they see a seizure. For many, the reaction of others to their epilepsy is worse than the seizures themselves. Rejection and exclusion can cause low self-esteem and low self-confidence.

HAVING BLANKET RULES FOR PEOPLE WITH EPILEPSY IS WRONG

There are many different types of epilepsy and very few rules that could reasonably apply to all people with seizures. For instance, contrary to what many people think, all people with epilepsy can watch TV and get involved in sports. If seizures are sometimes triggered by a standard TV, a "flicker-free" set (with a picture frequency of 100 Hz) or a flat screen TV can help. Seizures can also be avoided by not sitting too closely to the TV set.

Most people
with epilepsy may:

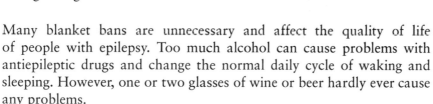

- drink moderate amounts of alcohol;
- go out on their own;
- play computer games;
- drive a car (if seizures are controlled);
- go to nightclubs.

Many blanket bans are unnecessary and affect the quality of life of people with epilepsy. Too much alcohol can cause problems with antiepileptic drugs and change the normal daily cycle of waking and sleeping. However, one or two glasses of wine or beer hardly ever cause any problems.

Risk should be assessed individually for each person. Everyone needs to discuss the risks that apply to them with their doctor or epilepsy nurse.

PEOPLE WITH EPILEPSY WANT TO LEAD A NORMAL LIFE

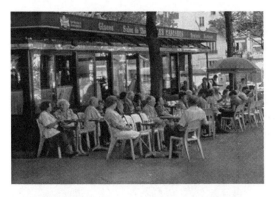

Most people with epilepsy would like to lead a perfectly normal life. However, some withdraw from others and become isolated because they feel rejected. The behavior of others toward people with epilepsy can cause emotional problems like depression. Some people with epilepsy find friendship and support in self-help groups.

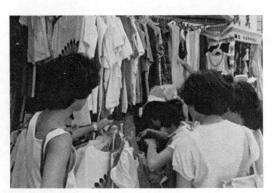

PEOPLE WITH EPILEPSY HAVE THE SAME RANGE OF INTELLIGENCE AS ANYONE ELSE

Some people with epilepsy are highly gifted; others are of average intelligence. In this respect they are no different from people without epilepsy. Because of this, there are children with epilepsy in all types of schools. Many people with seizures have completed a university degree and are very successful at work. People who have no health problem other than epilepsy can lead a normal life, both at home and at work, as long as those around them give them a chance to do so.

SAFETY IS A CONCERN FOR EVERYONE

People with epilepsy may need to take extra precautions: they may need to think of measures that reduce risks to themselves (for instance, related to falling or losing consciousness) and risks to others (for instance, small children in their care).

People who do not have seizures usually take it for granted that they will be safe in their home, at their workplace, when playing sports, or driving. For a person who has seizures, all of these places and situations may carry risks. However, the risk of injury can be reduced with small changes to a person's environment and to the way they normally do things.

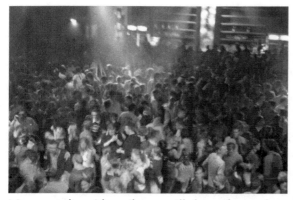

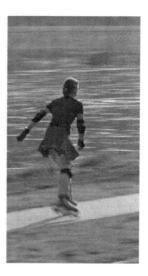

Most people with epilepsy will be safe in these situations.

Seizures that occur while driving or smoking can be disastrous not only for the person with epilepsy, but also for other people. Knowing the applicable law in your state and about when these activities are most dangerous can inform decisions about restrictions and precautions that can prevent accidents.

Safety measures for people with epilepsy should not only minimize injuries but also maximize the person's ability to lead a normal and active life.

SAFETY AT HOME

Most seizure-related accidents happen at home. Activities like bathing and cooking put people with seizures at risk of injury. Specific changes in the daily routine or environment can create a safer home. The particular type or nature of helpful adjustments depends on an individual's seizure type and frequency.

Bathrooms with large mirrors, shower doors, bathtubs, and hard floors can be risky for people with uncontrolled seizures.

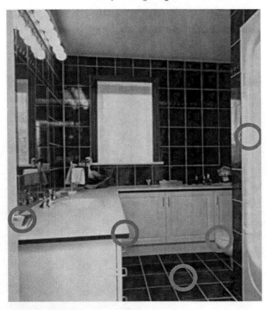

Circles indicate places where adjustments can be made to make this bathroom safer.

A few adjustments to the bathroom environment can make it safer for people with seizures. Shatterproof glass for mirrors and shower doors, as well as wall-to-wall carpeting, reduces the risk of injuries for individuals who fall during their seizures. Hanging the bathroom door so that it opens outwards (into the hall or bedroom) instead of inwards will allow helpers to enter the room even if the person has fallen against the door. Using protective covers on faucet handles, nozzles, and the edges of countertops can cushion falls and reduce injuries. It is a good safety strategy to avoid burns in the bathroom by covering the radiator or heating unit with a pad and to install safety devices that adjust water temperature.

Electrical equipment such as hair dryers or razors should not be used near a water source.

Example

Jenny, a 13-year-old girl with complex partial seizures was determined to maintain her independence and remain safe while using the bathroom. She negotiated with her parents that she would use an "occupied" sign instead of locking the bathroom door and sing in the shower to reassure her parents that she was safe. She also promised always to take showers instead of baths and to check the water temperature and shower drain before using the shower.

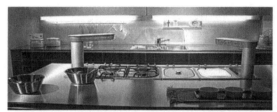
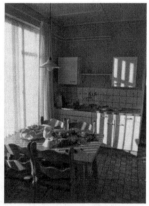
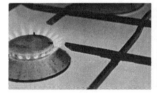
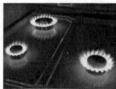

The kitchen, with its ovens, burners, and sharp knives is another area that holds potential hazards. Adjustments in the way food is prepared and cooked and in the way the kitchen and cooking utensils are cleaned can make the kitchen safer for people with seizures. For example, a man with occasional complex partial seizures does all his food preparation with food processors or choppers instead of a knife. He buys pre-cut vegetables and salad or ready-prepared meals when possible. The microwave oven is safer than a stove. He uses rubber gloves when he cleans the kitchen. Unbreakable dishes reduce the risk of cuts.

Strategies that prevent injuries at home allow people to be safe and independent.

SPORT IS FUN AND CAN HELP IN DIFFICULT TIMES

Participating in sports is fun and gives people the opportunity to enjoy themselves on their own or with others.

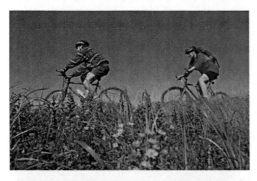

It can take one's mind off their problems and allow people to let off steam. This may be particularly important for people who have to live with a difficult medical condition.

Sports that make people get out of breath do not increase the risk of seizures. Unlike overbreathing during the EEG, increased breathing during sports only helps to provide the body with the oxygen it needs.

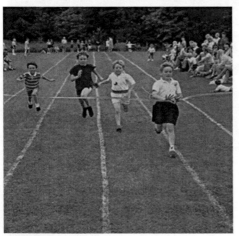

> People with epilepsy should not be banned from sports in general.

Serious injuries to people with epilepsy rarely occur during participation in sports. The bathroom is much more dangerous to a teen with epilepsy than the soccer field. Any decision should be based on common sense. The goals should be both safety and a lifestyle that is as normal as possible. No activity is completely safe. If in doubt, discuss particular types of sports with a doctor or nurse.

> Most people with epilepsy are able to enjoy sports.

MANY PEOPLE ENJOY THEIR SPORTS

For many people, sport is an important part of life. It helps them to stay fit and feel better about themselves. Very few people with epilepsy cannot take part in sports. There is no reason why children with epilepsy should be automatically banned from school sports. Sports clubs can make it easier to mix with others and can help people feel less isolated. Feeling better about themselves helps people to be more independent and to deal with their seizures. This can improve their quality of life and may also improve the seizures by lowering stress levels.

Teens with epilepsy are encouraged to participate in group and competitive sports such as league baseball, community sports, and varsity sports at school. These activities are usually well super-

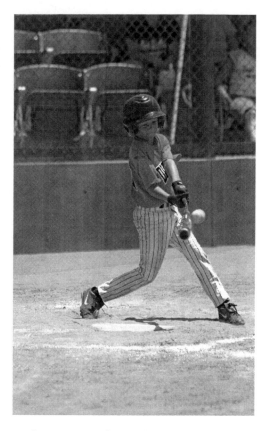

With permission from Alex Miroshnichenko, Miro-Foto

vised, and most teens with epilepsy can participate safely without special arrangements. In many cases, the risk may not be increased at all; for instance, if people have enough warning of their seizures to make sure that they are in a safe position or if seizures only happen during sleep. Some people have other problems in addition to epilepsy, like being a little slow or clumsy in their reactions. This should be taken into account when choosing a particular type of sport.

If in doubt about a sport, it is best to ask a doctor or nurse.

RISKS DEPEND ON THE TYPE OF EPILEPSY AND ON THE TYPE OF SPORT

Sports can cause injuries whether or not someone has epilepsy. In many types of sport (like badminton, dancing, or table tennis) the risk of injury is no greater for people who have seizures than for those without epilepsy. Other sports are more dangerous, for instance, if there is a risk of falling from a height or drowning. In such sports, people with epilepsy may need to be watched carefully by others, take special precautions (like wearing a crash-helmet), or they may be unable to do the sport altogether (like diving or shooting).

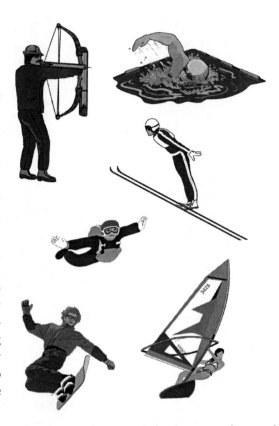

These types of sport may be dangerous for people with epilepsy.

If seizures are likely to happen, it is best to advise team members about them.

This gives them the opportunity to learn about epilepsy and to find out what to do in case of a seizure. Otherwise they may feel helpless and frightened if a seizure happens, and they may not do the right things.

Both the type of sport and the types of seizures should be considered in deciding whether a sport is suitable.

CHILDREN WITH EPILEPSY DEVELOP IN THE SAME WAY AS OTHER CHILDREN

Many children with epilepsy develop normally and do not need any particular support. However, there are some children who do not just have epilepsy but also other disorders of the brain. If children with epilepsy need extra help, it can be difficult to strike the right balance between supporting them and stopping them from becoming more independent. Children who receive too much attention can feel smothered and may not have much self-confidence.

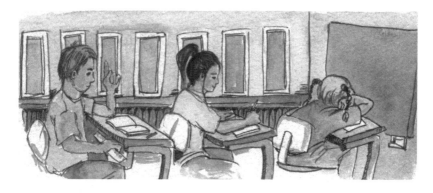

Epilepsy affects everyone in the family, not just the person with seizures. Reactions of family members to a diagnosis of epilepsy can range from denial to anger, fear, or acceptance. Not everyone in the family will feel the same thing.

When a child has been diagnosed with epilepsy, it is not a good idea to let this diagnosis take over the life of the whole family. On the other hand, members of the family have to give drugs regularly, help the child when there are seizures, keep a seizure diary, and go to the doctor's office or the hospital for follow-up visits. It is very difficult to find a middle way between seeming "careless" and being "overbearing." It may help to talk to other parents of children with epilepsy.

> Like everybody else, children with epilepsy have to be able to deal with problems and conflicts. They cannot learn this if they are always protected by their families and friends.

CHILDREN AND TEENAGERS WITH EPILEPSY CAN HAVE A HARD TIME

Young people with epilepsy do not only have to cope with increasing demands from their family and teachers at school, but also have to find ways of living with seizures and their treatment.

Being open about seizures helps teachers, school friends, family members, and neighbors to accept a child's epilepsy as part of normal life. Unfortunately, because many people know very little about epilepsy, they may be prejudiced against people who have seizures. Because of this, openness does not always work.

Still, it is generally much better if teachers and school friends know about epilepsy so that they do not get frightened by seizures and know what to do in the event of a seizure.

Parents of children with epilepsy often have a hard time.

Their child's future may seem uncertain. The child's epilepsy has an impact on many aspects of their lives. Sometimes the stress caused by this leads to friction between the parents. Parents should not hesitate to get advice from other parents of children with epilepsy, from a counselor, or a self-help group if they experience this sort of friction.

Self-help groups help with many family problems.

SMOKING IS A RISK FOR PEOPLE WITH AND WITHOUT EPILEPSY

Smoking tobacco is not known to have any definite effects on seizure control. But people with epilepsy are not only susceptible to all the usual effects of smoking but are also at increased risk of injury or death from fire. Unlike many other activities, smoking does represent a risk not only to the health of the person with epilepsy but also to others who may be harmed if a cigarette starts a fire during a seizure. Therefore, any person with epilepsy who blacks out in their seizures should seriously consider stopping smoking. Let your doctor know because the dose of your seizure medicine, especially phenytoin, may need to be lowered once you no longer smoke or take nicotine.

The use of nicotine patches to help break the smoking habit is safe for people with epilepsy. The use of Zyban (bupropion) tablets as an aid to stop smoking can increase the seizure frequency or intensity, but at the usual dosage of 300 mg per day, the risk of worsening the seizures is small.

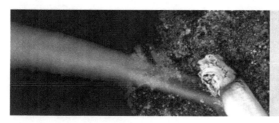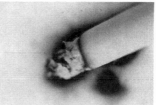

Example

A 35-year-old woman with absence and tonic-clonic seizures shared an apartment with her 5-year-old daughter. One evening, the woman had a tonic-clonic seizure while smoking. When she awoke in the hospital, she had first-degree burns on a large part of her arms and body. Her daughter suffered severe smoke inhalation and brain damage. The woman stopped smoking and was badly traumatized by this accident.

Smoking contributes to the death of approximately 500,000 people each year from heart disease, stroke, and cancer.

MANY PEOPLE WITH EPILEPSY LIKE TO TRAVEL

Short trips that do not cause any major changes to the daily routine cause few problems. Longer trips or long-distance travel, however, need to be planned more carefully. Are vaccinations needed? Is travel going to cause lack of sleep? Is the destination in a different time zone? If so, at what times should tablets be taken? Does the dose of the antiepileptic drugs have to be adjusted? How do you deal with diarrhea and vomiting if you have to take tablets?

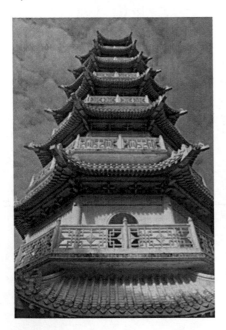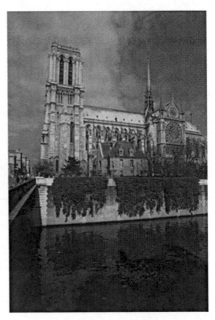

Travelers to some countries need to prepare for their trip by having vaccinations and by taking tablets before they leave to avoid getting diseases like malaria. However, some drugs that are used to prevent malaria are best avoided in people with epilepsy. Travelers to hot countries often develop diarrhea. Many people treat this sort of diarrhea with carbon tablets. This is not a good idea for people who have to take antiepileptic drugs, as the carbon tablets can reduce their effect. Another thing to think about is health insurance. In other countries, people may need additional travel health insurance.

LONGER TRIPS SHOULD BE DISCUSSED WITH A DOCTOR AND PLANNED IN ADVANCE

Long-distance travel is exhausting and tiring. It can upset the usual daily routine of being awake and being asleep. In some cases, tranquilizers (benzodiazepines) may be helpful. Traveling long distance with the sun (westwards) or against the sun (eastwards) is particularly difficult. Travel in these directions causes days to be unusually long or short. This means that it may be advisable to change the dose of antiepileptic drugs taken on the day of travel. People with epilepsy planning a flight east or west should discuss this with their doctor.

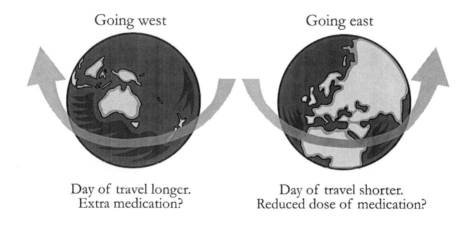

Going west

Going east

Day of travel longer.
Extra medication?

Day of travel shorter.
Reduced dose of medication?

Flying north or south causes fewer problems because this does not affect the normal daily rhythm. Slower modes of travel (like ships) cause less disruption than flying. People traveling by plane should keep all the medication needed for the vacation (and a few extra doses) in their hand luggage, so there is less risk of losing it. A doctor's letter might help to avoid problems at customs.

Extra doses of antiepileptic drugs may have to be taken in case of vomiting or diarrhea. It is unlikely, for instance, that the body would have taken up much of a drug if tablets are brought up within half an hour of taking the dose. In this case, it may be best to take a second dose. If possible though, advice should be sought from a doctor.

4.2 EPILEPSY AT SCHOOL AND AT WORK

TEACHERS SHOULD BE WELL INFORMED ABOUT EPILEPSY

Often epilepsy is first noticed at school. Teachers should know about three common types of seizures:

Absence seizures: These are brief lapses of consciousness. Children are often thought to be daydreaming at first, and not concentrating on their work. Each absence only lasts a few seconds but one absence seizure can quickly be followed by another.

Complex partial seizures: In these seizures, consciousness is often impaired for several minutes. People may seem to behave oddly, they may fiddle with their clothes, laugh for no reason, or smack their lips.

Generalized tonic-clonic seizures: This is the best-known type of seizure. The whole body stiffens and shakes. Consciousness only comes back very slowly.

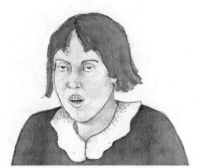

Absence seizure

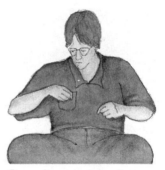

Complex partial seizure

Not every epileptic seizure is an emergency.

Seizures are not the fault of the teacher, the classmates, or the school. They are part of a disorder. A seizure can rarely be stopped or prevented (other than by taking daily medication). If a seizure occurs, it is important to stay calm. Almost all seizures stop on their own.

At school, children with epilepsy should be treated in the same way as other children.

WHAT TO DO IF A SEIZURE OCCURS AT SCHOOL

- Stay calm, the seizure cannot be stopped.
- Make sure the child having the seizure is safe.
- Keep an eye on the time.
- A seizure should not last longer than 5–10 minutes.
- Observe the seizure and offer help after it has passed.

In status epilepticus, an ambulance should be called.

In status epilepticus, one seizure is followed by another. It is a medical emergency and has to be treated without delay. Status may just consist of two major seizures in 1 hour without full recovery of consciousness in between. In more severe cases, major seizures may occur within minutes of each other.

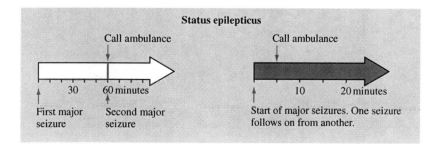

What Not to Do if a Seizure Occurs at School

- Panic
- Try to "wake up" the child having the seizure
- Try to stop the seizure
- Try to put antiepileptic drugs in the mouth
- Try to resuscitate during the seizure
- Put things in their mouth to stop people from "swallowing their tongue"
- Mouth-to-mouth breathing
- Hold the child down
- Leave the child alone
- Try to "wake up" the child from sleep after the seizure

Most seizures that happen at school are completely unpredictable. They may, however, be more likely with lack of sleep, stress, infections with high temperature, or on school trips.

PARENTS SHOULD TELL TEACHERS ABOUT THEIR CHILD'S EPILEPSY

When teachers know that a child has epilepsy, they can try to help. Teachers will understand that a child's performance can vary if antiepileptic drugs have to be changed. Teachers can also try to make sure that a child with epilepsy is accepted by their classmates and does not feel excluded.

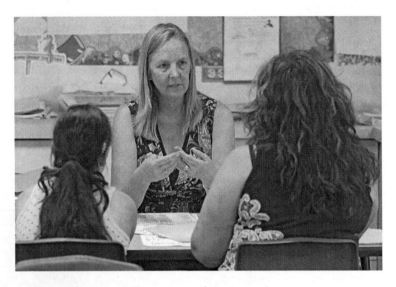

With permission from Denis Poroy: www.dpimages.us/

Most children with epilepsy are otherwise healthy. Often, the only thing they know about their seizures is how people around them react to the attacks. Poorly informed adults may react to seizures with fear or panic, which the children may not understand at all.

In some children, epileptic seizures are caused by other diseases, for instance disorders of the body's metabolism. Such children may have other problems as well as epilepsy.

> Children who only have epilepsy can do just as well at school as other children.

LIKE ALL STUDENTS, THOSE WITH EPILEPSY SHOULD FEEL SAFE AND ACCEPTED

Whether these goals are achieved depends on other people's understanding of epilepsy, their ability to respond to seizures, and their beliefs about the abilities of students with epilepsy.

Epilepsy education and awareness should be part of the school curriculum whenever one or more students at school have epilepsy. Because seizures are unpredictable, anyone at school may need to respond to a seizure. Epilepsy education usually involves bringing in outside speakers from a local Epilepsy Foundation affiliate or a nearby epilepsy center.

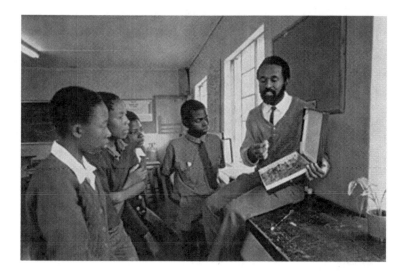

Ideally, epilepsy education should begin before there is a crisis at school, rather than after a seizure has caught everyone by surprise. Therefore, the parents of a child with epilepsy (or college students themselves) should consider notifying the school before classes start. Discussion of the best response to a seizure can be supplemented with specific instructions from the student's doctor and input from the school nurse and health educator.

Students with epilepsy face challenges unknown to other students.

EPILEPSY MAY NEED TO BE CONSIDERED WHEN CHOOSING A CAREER

People who have been free of seizures for many years can do almost any job. A small number of jobs are an exception to this. Even when people have been seizure-free for a number of years they may not be able to work as an airplane pilot or train driver, pilot, and soldier. People who are not free of seizures have to consider the risk to themselves and others that come with particular jobs. Jobs that involve using handheld or open machinery could put people at risk of injuring themselves.

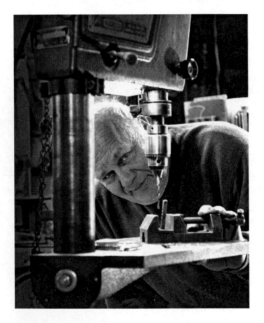

With permission from Chris Rioux: www.ChrisRiouxPhotography.com

The level of risk also depends on the type of seizures. For example, the risk would be lessened if someone always had sufficient warning before their seizures to step back from dangerous machinery. If seizures would cause an increased risk of harm to the worker or others, epilepsy should be discussed with the employer. Under the Americans with Disabilities Act, the employer is obliged to make reasonable adjustments to make the job safe. If the workplace cannot be made safe, the employer would be expected to try to find alternative employment in the same company.

The risk of injuries is often overestimated.

FINDING AND KEEPING A GOOD JOB CAN BE A CHALLENGE

Having a job is important for raising self-esteem, supporting a family, and affording health insurance. However, unemployment rates among people with epilepsy are higher than for the general population. Seizures or side effects from medication can make it difficult to complete as much school or job training as one would like. If driving is not allowed because of seizures, lack of transportation reduces the chance of finding a job. Employers give many different reasons for not hiring a person with epilepsy: These include concerns about safety, worry about the company's liability, concerns about the ability to function at the job, and fear that a seizure will scare off customers.

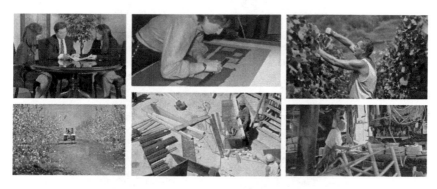

It can help people first to assess their qualifications, strengths, and weaknesses with a vocational counselor who has experience with epilepsy. Local public service groups may offer transportation for people who can't drive. Social workers or job counselors know what is available in the area. Sometimes people will need to consider moving for a job. Some good jobs can be done from home. Sometimes, it is possible to educate employers and co-workers. The Epilepsy Foundation or local epilepsy center may offer educational opportunities or brochures with further information.

> Most people with epilepsy are capable of having fulfilling jobs.

PEOPLE WITH EPILEPSY CAN WORK JUST AS HARD AS ANYONE ELSE

Many people with epilepsy are doing low-skilled jobs although they may be capable of doing higher-skilled work. This is true despite the fact that people with epilepsy are no more likely to be involved in a work-related accident than others.

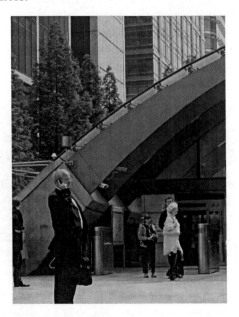

With permission from Andreas Hunziker, Switzerland, 2008

The problems people with epilepsy can face at work are mostly due to prejudice and misunderstanding. Because of this, it is sometimes better not to mention epilepsy when there have been no seizures for a long time. There is no obligation to mention epilepsy at a job interview unless it would significantly interfere with carrying out the principal work-related activities. However, people have to be honest about epilepsy when they undergo a medical check before they start a job or to find out whether they are able to continue doing their job. A job offer can only be withdrawn or people can only lose their job because of epilepsy if the seizures make it impossible for someone to do their job safely.

> Many people with epilepsy have unjustified difficulties at work because of epilepsy.

4.3   EPILEPSY AND PREGNANCY

MANY PEOPLE WITH EPILEPSY WANT TO HAVE A PARTNER AND A FAMILY

Whether to marry or to have children are personal decisions that everybody should make for themselves. However, people with epilepsy may be able to avoid problems and reduce risks if they are well informed about their condition and its treatment.

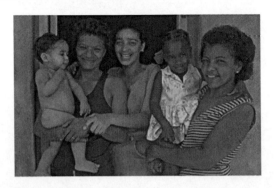

Things that may be considered when starting a relationship and a family:

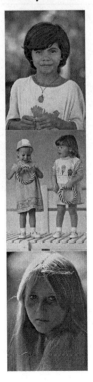

- There is no reason to rush into the disclosure of epilepsy. Unless seizures are so frequent that one might occur on the first date, it is best to wait until the ice is broken and trust and openness have developed in the relationship. If this trust does not develop, the relationship should probably not go any further and the diagnosis of epilepsy will not need to be discussed. If the relationship is promising, it may be a good idea to discuss the epilepsy earlier rather than later. It is best to tell the other person face to face, not over the telephone or by letter. A successful partnership is based on openness.

- Anyone who dates and gets involved in romantic relationships is likely to experience rejection at some time or other. Some prospective partners may say no to the first date or the second date, and others break up the relationship after an extended period of dating. Rejection is, unfortunately, part of dating and relationships for everyone; it is not unique to people with epilepsy.

- Having a partner who also has epilepsy can improve mutual understanding. However, the risk of having children with epilepsy is higher if both parents have epilepsy.

- People with epilepsy can generally enjoy the same sexual feelings and pleasures as anyone else. Epilepsy is not generally associated with restrictions on sexual activities. Most people with epilepsy have normal sex lives. There is no convincing evidence that seizures are more likely to occur during sexual activities.

- Many antiepileptic drugs (like carbamazepine, phenytoin, and topiramate) reduce the strength of the oral contraceptive pill; others do not (like valproate, gabapentin, and levetiracetam). Bleeding between periods is a sure sign that the oral contraceptive pill is not providing enough protection and higher doses or other forms of contraception (like condoms) should be used under the guidance of a physician.

- Pregnancy should be planned well in advance. It is a good idea to think about childcare and how children will be looked after, so that they will not be at risk of injury if one of their parents has a seizure.

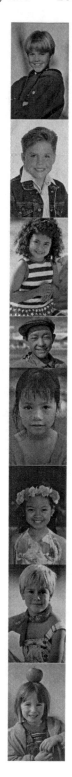

PEOPLE WITH EPILEPSY HAVE A SLIGHTLY HIGHER RISK OF HAVING CHILDREN WITH EPILEPSY

The chance of having a child with epilepsy depends on the type of the father's or mother's epilepsy. On average, the risk is around 3 percent. If both parents have epilepsy, the risk of children developing epilepsy is considerably higher.

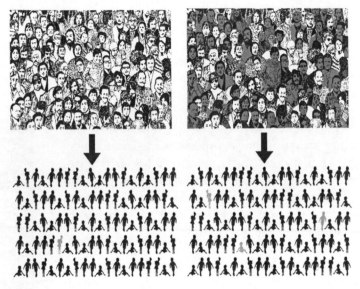

The picture gives an idea of the level of the risk. The left side shows that 1 out of 100 children born to parents without epilepsy will develop epilepsy. The right side shows what happens when one of the parents has epilepsy. Even so, 97 out of 100 children will not have epilepsy.

If children born to parents with epilepsy develop epilepsy themselves, it is often the same type as their parents'. If, for instance, the father or mother developed absence seizures around the age of 9, it is most likely that the child will also have absences (if they develop epilepsy at all). Epilepsy does not get worse by being passed on from parents to their children.

ANTIEPILEPTIC DRUGS CAN DAMAGE BABIES IN THE WOMB

However, the risk of antiepileptic drugs is much lower than often thought.

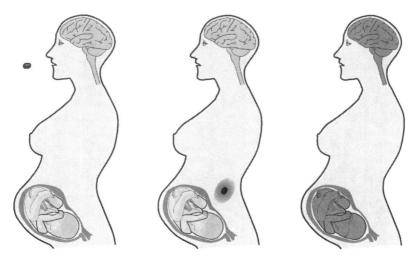

The drugs are taken up by the blood of the mother. The baby in the womb is fed by the mother's blood. If antiepileptic drugs are carried by the blood, they can also reach the baby. All drugs have the potential to harm a baby in the womb. However, stopping antiepileptic drugs could cause a dangerous increase of the number of seizures or status epilepticus. This would be a serious risk to the health of the mother and, indirectly, to the health of the baby. During pregnancy the number of seizures can increase. However, some women also have fewer seizures. We do not fully understand how and why pregnancy can have different effects on epilepsy in different women, but it is important to visit your doctor more frequently during pregnancy and have more frequent blood tests to monitor the levels of your seizure medicines.

> **Pregnancy causes a small increase of the risk of developing status epilepticus.**

MOTHERS WITH EPILEPSY HAVE A SLIGHTLY HIGHER RISK OF HAVING CHILDREN WITH ABNORMALITIES

Abnormalities are caused by problems with the development of the baby's body or organs. Examples of abnormalities include holes in the heart, or poor development of part of the face or the backbone.

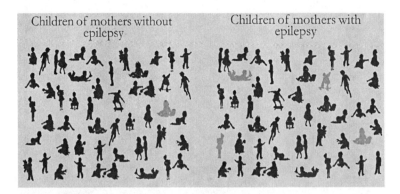

Children of mothers without epilepsy   Children of mothers with epilepsy

Parents without epilepsy can also have children with abnormalities.

The picture shows that 1 out of 50 children born to mothers without epilepsy has an abnormality. Among mothers with epilepsy, abnormalities are found in 4 out of 50 children (shown on the right). These numbers include relatively small abnormalities like a slightly widened bridge of the nose. Severe abnormalities are less common.

Most abnormalities are caused by antiepileptic drugs. However, there is some evidence that seizures (especially status epilepticus) can also damage babies in the womb.

> It can be dangerous to stop taking antiepileptic drugs out of concern about abnormalities! Medication changes are best discussed with and managed by a doctor.

THE RISK OF ABNORMALITIES CAN BE REDUCED IF PREGNANCY IS PLANNED IN ADVANCE

The baby's organs are formed in the first weeks and months of pregnancy. This is the time when abnormalities can develop.

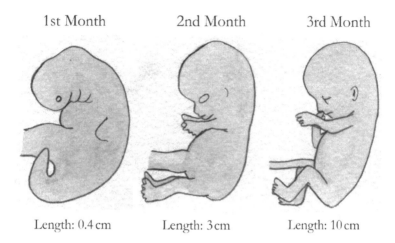

1st Month   2nd Month   3rd Month

Length: 0.4 cm   Length: 3 cm   Length: 10 cm

It is best to talk to a doctor before conception to see how the risk of abnormalities can be reduced. There are a number of things that may be done:

- In certain cases, drugs may be lowered or withdrawn completely.
- Treatment may be changed from several drugs to one.
- It may be possible to lower the dose.
- It may be better to take several doses a day or switch to slow-release drugs.
- The diet may be improved to increase the intake of folic acid (at least 0.4 mg/day), and other vitamins may be recommended.

Pregnancy is best planned well in advance.

SERIOUS ABNORMALITIES CAN BE DISCOVERED DURING PREGNANCY

Many serious problems with a baby's development can be picked up with an ultrasound examination. If a severe abnormality is found, further options can be discussed. In some cases, abnormalities can be treated with surgery once the baby has been born. In some cases, parents may think about having an abortion.

ABNORMALITIES CAUSING LIFELONG DISABILITY ARE VERY RARE

Severe abnormalities often affect the heart, the brain, or the spinal cord. Comparatively minor abnormalities (such as widely spaced eyes, a small nose which points upwards, short fingers and toes) are more common.

MOST SEIZURES DO NOT AFFECT THE DEVELOPING BABY

A large number of major seizures (tonic-clonic) and status epilepticus are an exception. Status epilepticus can harm both mother and baby. There is no evidence that a single seizure affects the baby. It is not easy to weigh the risks from antiepileptic drugs against the risks of having major seizures. It is best if this issue is discussed with an epilepsy specialist before pregnancy and if epilepsy is treated by a specialist during pregnancy.

WOMEN WITH EPILEPSY CAN GIVE BIRTH IN THE NORMAL WAY

Few women experience seizures during labor, although the risk of having a seizure is higher than usual around the time of delivery. It is important to try to take the antiepileptic drug in the usual way. Babies born to mothers taking certain antiepileptic drugs, which speed up the way the liver works, should be given an injection of vitamin K because there is a slightly higher risk of bleeding.

ANTIEPILEPTIC DRUGS ARE ALSO FOUND IN BREAST MILK

Although antiepileptic drugs can be found in breast milk, the doses in the milk are usually so low that they do no harm to the baby. Breast milk also contains all the nourishment a baby needs and it strengthens the baby's defense system against infections. If the mother takes large doses of phenobarbital, primidone, or benzodiazepines (for instance diazepam or clonazepam) as treatment for epilepsy, the drugs in the breast milk can cause babies to be sleepy and to suck poorly. If this happens, mothers can switch to bottle feeding altogether, or they can try a mixture of breast- and bottle-feeding.

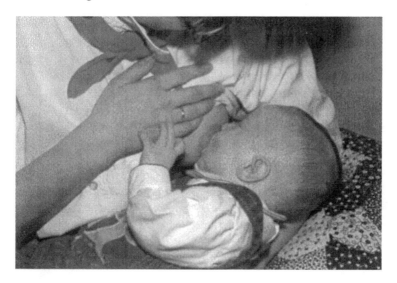

A child does not just bring joy but also stress and change. Often regular and sufficient sleep can only be guaranteed if both parents help, for instance when looking after the baby during the night. Breast milk can be pumped off so that the father can bottle-feed at night. If people have seizures that could put them at risk of dropping their baby, it may also be best for someone without epilepsy to bathe the baby.

> Most women with epilepsy can breast-feed even if they are taking drugs to stop their seizures.

FDA (FOOD AND DRUG ADMINISTRATION) PREGNANCY CATEGORIES

Women who are pregnant or considering pregnancy are rightly concerned about whether the medicines they take might cause birth defects or other harm to their developing baby. The Food and Drug Administration is one source of guidance. The FDA looks at the evidence available about the risk of harm if each medication is used during pregnancy. Then it assigns each one to a "Pregnancy Category" (A, B, C, D, or X). The category for each medication is reported in its package insert.

Category

A Adequate, well/controlled studies in pregnant women have not shown any risk to the fetus in the first 3 months of pregnancy, and there is no evidence of later risk either. No antiepileptic drugs have been assigned to this level.

B Studies using animals have not found any risk to the fetus, or animal studies that have found risk were not confirmed by adequate studies in pregnant women.

C Studies using animals have shown a harmful effect on the fetus, or there haven't been any studies in either women or animals. Caution is advised, but the benefits of the medication may outweigh the potential risks.

D There is clear evidence of risk to the human fetus, but the benefits may outweigh the risk for pregnant women who have a serious condition that cannot be treated effectively with a safer drug.

X There is clear evidence that the medication causes abnormalities in the fetus. The risks outweigh any potential benefits for women who are (or may become) pregnant.

4.4 EPILEPSY AND THE LAW

EVERYONE IS EQUAL BEFORE THE LAW

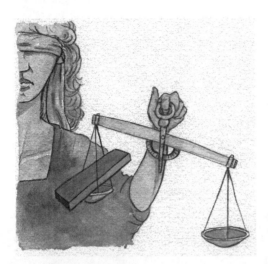

People with epilepsy should not have to face unfair discrimination because of their epilepsy. However, there are some situations in which people with epilepsy are not treated in the same way as others. People can only fight for their rights if they know what their rights are. Epilepsy can be an issue in legal disputes with employers or with insurance companies.

A child who "only" has epilepsy should go to a mainstream nursery and school.

Children with epilepsy without any additional learning disabilities or medical conditions have the same range of intelligence and abilities as children without epilepsy. Children with epilepsy and other conditions who need extra provision can have their needs met through the "Individuals with Disabilities Education Act." For this reason, the majority of children with epilepsy are educated in mainstream schools or nurseries.

The Americans with Disabilities Act covers children with epilepsy. This means that they have the same rights to attend the school of their choice as other children. Should a school refuse a child with epilepsy a place, this could be considered discriminatory. Unless there is absolutely no "reasonable adjustment" that the school could make to accommodate the child, the school's refusal of a place because of epilepsy is against the law.

EDUCATION SHOULD MATCH A CHILD'S NEEDS

The Individuals with Disabilities Education Act (IDEA) requires public schools to make available to all eligible children with disabilities a free appropriate public education in the least restrictive environment appropriate to their individual needs. IDEA requires public school systems to develop individualized education programs for each child. IDEA also mandates that particular procedures be followed in the development of the education program. Each program must be developed by a team of knowledgeable persons and must be reviewed at least annually. The team includes the child's teacher, the parents (subject to certain limited exceptions), the child (if determined appropriate), an agency representative, and other individuals at the parents' or agency's discretion.

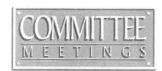 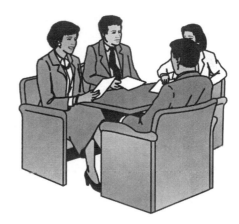

If parents disagree with the proposed individualized education program, they can request a due-process hearing and a review from the state educational agency if applicable in that state. They also can appeal the state agency's decision to state or federal court.

You are your child's greatest advocate.

PEOPLE WITH EPILEPSY ARE ONLY LIABLE FOR DAMAGE CAUSED BY A SEIZURE IF THEY WERE NEGLIGENT

It is very unusual that someone has to pay for damage caused by a seizure, although they could be held responsible if they had been negligent. As an example, someone with epilepsy may have to pay for damage caused during a seizure in a nightclub if they knew in advance that the flashing lights would cause a seizure and that there would be flashing lights inside the nightclub. Liability insurance may not have to pay for damage if it occurred because the insured person was "negligent" or careless.

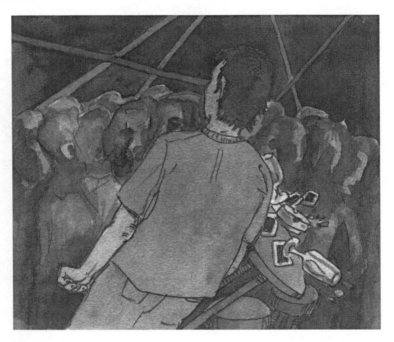

A person with epilepsy would not have to pay for the damage if they had not known that flashing lights would trigger a seizure. Someone who has never had seizures before is not usually responsible for any damage caused in a first seizure.

INSURANCE COMPANIES OFTEN WANT TO KNOW WHEN EPILEPSY BEGAN

Insurance companies are always interested in reducing their risk. If an insurance company can prove that an illness or medical condition increases the risk that they may have to pay out, the premium will be higher or a policy may be refused altogether. Many insurance application forms ask about chronic illness or medical conditions. People who do not tell the truth on an application form may find that they have no coverage if they try to submit a claim, even if they have paid their premiums on time. Some insurance policies also state that the person who has taken out the insurance has to inform the insurance company about changes in their health status. For instance, people who are first diagnosed with epilepsy may have to inform a private health, car, or life insurance company of their condition.

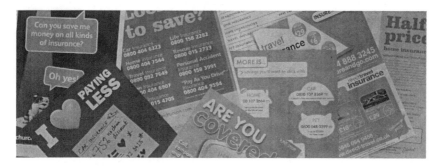

It can be difficult for people with epilepsy to get private health insurance. If epilepsy is diagnosed after health insurance has been taken out, the insurance company will not be able to increase the premium or refuse coverage. Some insurance companies will try to exclude any claims caused by epilepsy. Sometimes such exclusions actually break the law. Self-help groups, disabled rights groups, or a disability lawyer may be able to help.

> It can be a good idea to maintain insurance coverage that was arranged before epilepsy was diagnosed.

BASIC RIGHTS OF PEOPLE WITH DISABILITIES ARE DEFINED BY THE AMERICANS WITH DISABILITIES ACT (ADA)

Since 1990, the ADA has provided a clear and comprehensive set of rules about discrimination on the basis of disability. Protection for persons with epilepsy was further strengthened by the ADA Amendments Act of 2008.

"A Guide to Disability Rights Laws" has been created by the Disability Rights Section of the U.S. Department of Justice and can be downloaded from: http://www.ada.gov/cguide.pdf

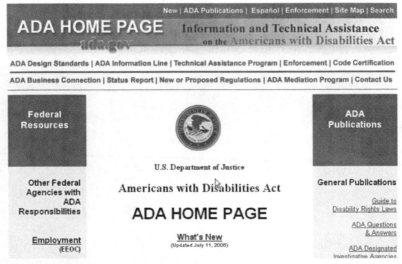

http://www.usdoj.gov/crt/ada

In order to be protected by the ADA, you must meet certain criteria. To be protected by the ADA, one must have a disability or have a relationship or association with an individual with a disability. The ADA defines a person with a disability as one who has physical or mental impairments that substantially limit one or more major life activities, a person who has a history or record of such an impairment, or a person who is perceived by others as having such an impairment. The ADA does not specifically name all of the impairments that are covered.

ADA MEDIATION PROGRAM

Mediation is an informal process in which an impartial third party helps disputing parties to find mutually satisfactory solutions to their differences. Mediation can resolve disputes quickly and satisfactorily, without the expenses and delay of formal investigation and litigation. Mediation proceedings are confidential and voluntary for all parties. Mediation typically involves one or more meetings between the disputing parties and the mediator. Mediators are *not* judges. Their role is to manage the process through which parties resolve their conflict. The mediators in the Department of Justice program are professionals who have been trained in the legal requirements of the ADA.

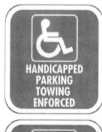
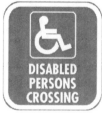
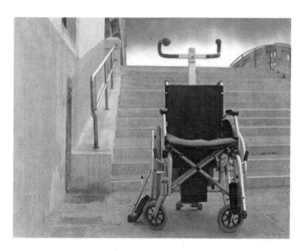

To work with a mediator, one must file a complaint with the Department and note on the complaint form that the dispute should be taken to mediation.

The ADA prohibits discrimination on the basis of disability in employment, state and local governments, public accommodations, commercial facilities, transportation, and telecommunications.

EMPLOYMENT DISCRIMINATION ON THE BASIS OF EPILEPSY IS ILLEGAL

Employers with 15 or more employees have to provide qualified individuals with disabilities an equal opportunity to benefit from the full range of employment-related opportunities available to others. For example, the Americans with Disabilities Act prohibits discrimination in:

→ Recruitment
→ Hiring
→ Promotions
→ Training
→ Pay
→ Social activities

Complaints must be filed with the U.S. Equal Employment Opportunity Commission (EEOC) within 180 days of the date of discrimination, or 300 days if the charge is filed with a designated State or local fair employment practice agency.

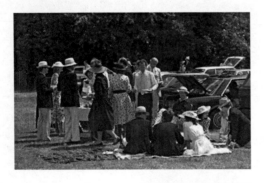

When a charge is filed, EEOC informs the employer within 10 days. Charges are given the most prompt attention when the facts seem to show that it is likely that discrimination has occurred. If discrimination is found, EEOC will seek a remedy for the charging party through conciliation.

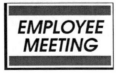

Was this meeting available for all employees?

DO EMPLOYERS HAVE TO BE TOLD ABOUT EPILEPSY?

There are very few jobs people with epilepsy are not allowed to do at all, for instance being an airline pilot or train driver. It is all right not to mention epilepsy at an interview for a job or on a job application form if an epileptic seizure in the workplace would cause no more harm to yourself or to others than when at home or while out and about. This may be particularly appropriate if seizures have been fully controlled for months or years.

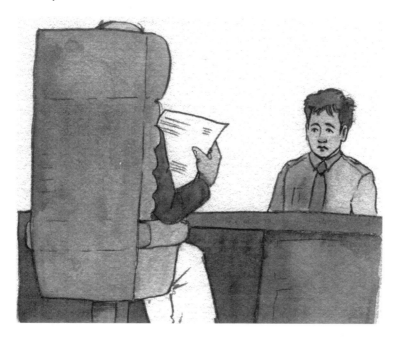

However, people should be honest about epilepsy when they undergo a work-related medical check, for instance before they start a job. People also have to inform the employer about their epilepsy if their seizures could cause harm at a workplace. Depending on the seizure type and job, it may be possible to make the workplace safe. The employer or the union may have ideas about how this can be done. If you decide to talk to an employer about epilepsy, it is best to be as matter-of-fact about your seizures as possible. It may be a good idea to practice this in advance, for instance with friends. You could also ask your doctor to write a letter about your epilepsy for your employer.

AN EPILEPTIC SEIZURE WHILE DRIVING A CAR CAN BE VERY DANGEROUS

People who experience seizures that alter awareness, consciousness, or muscle control may not be allowed to drive. Each state has its own regulations. The driving laws for all states relating to epilepsy can be found at http://www.epilepsy.com/epilepsy/rights_driving.html.

The laws in all 50 states restrict driver's licenses if seizures are not controlled by medication and establish rules regarding when and how a license may be acquired. Typically, a person has to be seizure-free for a specified period of time, commonly 6 months, and have a physician's statement confirming that the individual's seizures are controlled and that, if the person is licensed to drive, they will not present an unreasonable risk to public safety.

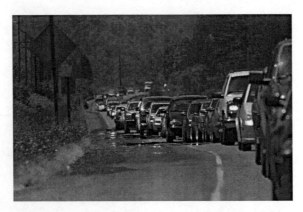

With permission from Jennifer Schmidt

These regulations are not completely satisfactory because they do not take into account that seizures affect different people in different ways. Obviously, it would be unsafe for someone who has major seizures without warning to drive. But what about people who only have seizures that cause twitching in one hand? They are banned because small seizures have the potential to develop into major seizures. But not all people with angina are banned from driving because they are at risk of heart attacks.

Very few accidents are caused by epileptic seizures.

5

CONDITIONS ASSOCIATED WITH EPILEPSY

DISORDERS THAT CAN BE ASSOCIATED WITH EPILEPSY

Some people with epilepsy also have other medical disorders. These other disorders may be completely unrelated to their epilepsy. On the other hand, epilepsy can be the cause of an additional disorder or the consequence of another health problem.

Sometimes, epileptic seizures are the first sign of another condition or disease.

This chapter will first focus on health problems that can be caused by epilepsy. The second part of the chapter describes other disorders or conditions that can cause epileptic seizures and epilepsy.

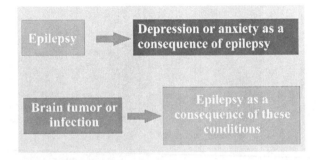

When a medical disorder causes epileptic seizures, doctors do not always make a diagnosis of epilepsy. If people have seizures that were clearly provoked by another disorder (for instance, a low sodium level caused by diuretic medication—water tablets), treatment should involve the removal of the underlying cause of the seizures and not antiepileptic drugs. However, other medical conditions associated with epilepsy may not always be cured as easily, and people's quality of life may then be affected by two chronic disorders.

MANY PEOPLE WITH EPILEPSY HAVE SYMPTOMS OF DEPRESSION

Everyone feels sad from time to time. When sadness is prolonged and impairs a person's ability to lead his/her life, he/she may be depressed. However, it may be difficult to distinguish clearly between the kind of sadness that is quite natural if someone has had a difficult time and the kind of low mood that might be considered a form of depression.

Only a qualified mental health professional, such as a psychiatrist or psychologist, should diagnose psychological problems. Self-diagnosis is not recommended. The information provided here is intended to help to determine whether you or a friend or a family member should consult a specialist for an evaluation and treatment. The information provided here is general and simplified. When you would like to talk to someone who can help with depression, consult your doctor, epilepsy nurse, or a psychologist.

Epilepsy can be the cause of depression. About one to two in five people with epilepsy have signs of depression. Identifying depression is particularly important in people with epilepsy because antiepileptic drugs can make depression worse and have been shown to increase the risk of suicide.

Depression may not be recognized during a routine office visit. Because of the time constraints, the seizure frequency is often the main focus of the conversation with the doctor. However, it has been shown that the frequency of their seizures has a smaller effect on people's quality of life than depression or anxiety.

IT IS IMPORTANT TO RECOGNIZE DEPRESSION

Sadness is common and natural. It is part of the spectrum of normal emotions that everybody experiences. However, when it is persistent, excessive, and affects other aspects of the way we think, it may become a problem. It is then called "depression" to distinguish it from "normal" sadness. It is important to recognize and address depression because it can have such a profound impact on people's quality of life.

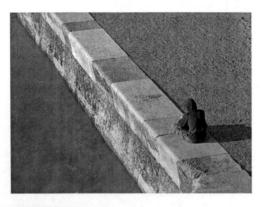

With permission from Frances Ellen Pe-Aguirre (http://frances.effronte.org)

The most important signs of depression are as follows:

- Lack of pleasure from activities that previously brought enjoyment
- Difficulties with concentration and making decisions
- Lack of patience and snappiness
- Decreased energy
- Tiredness
- Problems with sleep
- Changes in appetite
- Problems with weight
- Feeling hopeless
- Feeling worthless
- Feeling guilty
- Frequent thoughts of suicide and death

People with depression will experience several of these signs over days, weeks, or even years. There are a number of different forms of depression. In some people with epilepsy, signs of depression are clearly linked to their seizures. For instance, depression may precede a seizure by several hours or days. Brief periods of profound depression or panic can also be part of the seizure itself. Signs of depression are most common after seizures. Some people experience depression in between seizures, but their signs of depression clear a few days before they have a seizure.

DEPRESSIVE DISORDERS COME IN DIFFERENT FORMS

Reactive depression

This is also called "adjustment disorder." It is recognized when signs of depression have developed in response to a clear stress like a new "diagnosis of epilepsy" or finding out that epilepsy surgery has not stopped seizures completely. Reactive depression is expected to resolve within 6 months of the stressful experience. This time-limited form of depression can develop into a more persistent type of depression, such as "dysthymic disorder" or "major depression."

Dysthymic disorder

This term refers to a low to moderate level of depression that persists for at least 2 years. Therefore, this form of depression is more enduring than reactive depression and more resistant to treatment. Some people with dysthymic disorder develop major depression at some time during the course of their depression.

Major depression

This is the most serious type of depression. People with this form of depression are likely to experience most of the typical signs of depression. However, there are important differences in the nature and severity of the signs different people with major depression notice. You do not need to feel suicidal to have a major depression.

Some people experience periods with signs of depression that alternate with periods when they are particularly energetic and optimistic. Feeling like this can also be a part of the normal spectrum of human emotions. Some people, however, become energetic to the extent that they are restless, or cannot sleep, or concentrate. They may engage in high-risk behaviors, develop feelings of exaggerated self-importance, or develop an unusual interest in sex. These are features of mania, and their combination with signs of depression is called bipolar disorder or manic-depressive illness.

DEPRESSION CAN MAKE EPILEPSY WORSE

Several scientific studies have examined the ways in which epilepsy and depression affect each other. In one study, 43 of 100 people with epilepsy experienced signs of depression after their seizures; 18 of these 43 people had several signs of depression lasting for more than 24 hours. During this time, they felt like people with major depression feel. Thirteen had suicidal thoughts. Most of the people who reported signs of depression also experienced anxiety, problems with sleep, and changes in appetite. Often, these problems had a greater impact on their life than the seizures themselves.

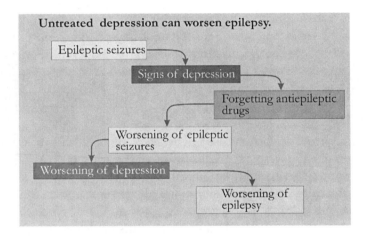

It is important for people with epilepsy who have additional signs of depression to get effective treatment for both the epilepsy and depression. Depression can be treated successfully with psychological treatment or antidepressant drugs.

Better recognition and treatment of depression have helped to reduce the suicide rate of people with epilepsy. It has declined by nearly one-third since 1990.

DEPRESSION IN CHILDREN AND TEENS WITH EPILEPSY

Depression is quite common in children and teens with epilepsy. Often children do not discuss their emotions openly with their parents. This means that parents have to be very aware of the signs of depression. If parents become concerned about depression, they can try to ask their children about any concerns or problems they have. Sometimes it may be easier for a specialist to receive answers to these questions.

A Number of Signs Can Indicate That a Child Is Depressed. The Child May...

- look anxious or unhappy.
- feel fearful, hopeless, lonely, rejected or guilty.
- become unusually quiet and withdraw from friends.
- have difficulties with concentration.
- keep mulling over negative thoughts.
- begin to do badly at school.
- complain of headaches or other pains.
- develop eating problems.
- have little energy or motivation to do anything.
- cry easily.
- be unusually aggressive or angry.

Some antiepileptic drugs can cause or increase depression. Sometimes parents contribute to a child's depression inadvertently although they are just trying to help. Children may feel robbed of their independence by parents trying to protect them. Parents who have low expectations of their children can reduce their children's self-esteem. Secrecy about epilepsy can cause children to be ashamed of their disorder. Most children are unlikely to realize that they are depressed themselves. This means that it is important to seek specialist advice early.

There are major differences between depression in children and in adults.

DEPRESSION CAN BE TREATED

Depression can be treated with different forms of psychological treatment (psychotherapy or talking treatment) or medication. It is important to know that the effect of antidepressant drugs is often delayed by 2–8 weeks. This means that the medication has to be taken regularly although people begin to feel better only after some time has passed while taking the medication.

There are several classes of drugs for depression. They differ in terms of their mode of action, side effects, and effects on epilepsy.

Amitriptyline, imipramine, nortriptyline, desipramine, trimipramine (tricyclic antidepressants, TCAs)

Used for depression for about 50 years; well-proven efficacy; common side effects include: sedation, low blood pressure, dry mouth, constipation, blurred vision. In overdose, they can cause death through effects on the heart; they can depress breathing and (especially in higher amounts) cause convulsions.

Fluoxetine, paroxetine, sertraline, citalopram, fluvoxamine (selective serotonin reuptake inhibitors, SSRIs)

These drugs are as effective as TCAs but cause side effects less frequently. They are unlikely to cause death in overdose and rarely cause epileptic seizures or a worsening of epilepsy.

Venlafaxine (serotonin and noradrenaline reuptake inhibitor, SNRI)

May be more useful in severe depressive illness and in depressions that are resistant to other drugs; possible side effects include an increase in blood pressure, severe agitation, headache, nausea. There is a small risk of making seizures worse.

Nefazodone (serotonin 2 antagonist/reuptake inhibitor)

Useful in people not tolerating SSRIs. Sometimes it induces anxiety, and people may complain of agitation when they start taking nefazodone.

Mirtazapine (noradrenergic and specific serotonergic antidepressant)

Useful when sedation is required in panic disorders or when depression is complicated by anxiety. Weight gain may be a problem.

Phenelzine, tranyecypromine (Monoamine oxidase inhibitors, MAOIs)

These drugs are used in unusual forms of depressions characterized by excessive eating or increased sexual activity. They are rarely used today. MAOIs should not be combined with other drugs against depression. People taking MAOIs have to avoid food that includes tyramine (like cheese).

Moclobemide (selective reversible inhibitor of monoamine oxidase, type A)

Works in a similar way to MAOIs, but is associated with fewer side effects or dietary problems. May not be useful in severe depression.

Medication for depression should be continued for 6–12 months even if the signs of depression resolve more quickly. It is important not to stop them suddenly because some can cause withdrawal reactions often involving panic and agitation.

Antidepressant drugs should not be thought of as a form of treatment that is likely to fix depression on its own. Increased physical activity can also reduce anxiety and improve physical health. Cognitive therapy targets depressive thinking patterns. Interpersonal therapy targets problems in relationships that may contribute to depression. Alcohol and recreational drugs can make depression worse and are probably best avoided.

EPILEPSY IS OFTEN ASSOCIATED WITH ANXIETY

Some people with epilepsy experience panic and fear as part of their seizures. In this case, the signs are caused by epileptic discharges in the brain. It may be difficult to distinguish between epileptic seizures causing panic feelings and panic attacks which appear as part of an anxiety disorder. Antiepileptic drug treatment would not help in people with anxiety disorder with the exception of benzodiazepines. The following features may help to make the distinction between panic in epileptic seizures and panic disorder.

Features of Anxiety as Part of Seizure versus Features of Anxiety in Panic Disorder

Anxiety as part of a seizure	Anxiety in a panic disorder
Lasts less than 30 seconds	Usually lasts several minutes
Intense fear or sensation of doom unlikely	Intense fear, sensation of "impending doom"
Fear may be followed by loss of awareness of surroundings	Intense sensation of doom may prevent detailed awareness of surroundings
Automatisms, no memory of this period	No clear memory gaps
Person may not be responsive to other people	Person remains responsive to other people

Anxiety is also quite common in between seizures. This form of anxiety can cause panic attacks, constant worrying, and fear of leaving the house or being left alone. Anxiety often occurs together with depression or disturbances of sleep and changes in appetite. Anxiety can be treated with the same drugs that can help with depression. Psychological treatment may also help.

Anxiety can reduce quality of life.

SEIZURES FOLLOWING METABOLIC DISORDERS

All parts of the body are constantly being broken down and rebuilt by chemical processes. The combination of all these chemical processes is the body's metabolism. Some aspects of metabolism are well understood.

Brain cells, for instance, need a constant supply of sugar. To achieve this supply, the amount of sugar in the blood is carefully controlled by the body. If the amount of sugar in the blood falls, the cells in the liver release sugar. If the sugar stores in the liver are exhausted or the liver does not release enough sugar, the levels of sugar become abnormally low. This state is called "hypoglycemia" and can cause epileptic seizures.

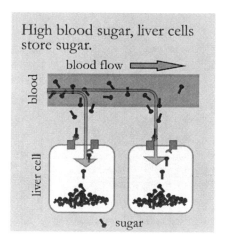 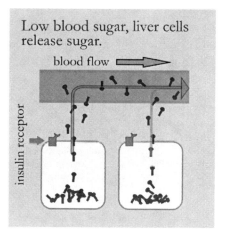

Seizures can also be caused by abnormally high blood sugar levels, for instance in severe forms of diabetes. If seizures are related to problems with the body's metabolism, it is essential to correct these problems quickly. Conventional antiepileptic drugs may not work. For this reason the blood sugar level is checked if someone is admitted to the hospital with a seizure. If the blood sugar is too high or too low, it can be corrected.

ABNORMAL BLOOD LEVELS OF SODIUM, MAGNESIUM, OR CALCIUM CAN CAUSE EPILEPTIC SEIZURES

Sodium, magnesium, and calcium are chemical constituents of different types of salts. They are very important for the functioning of nerve cells in the brain. The brain can only work properly if the levels of sodium, magnesium, and calcium are exactly right. Several organs of the body ensure that the blood levels do not change.

Sodium

About one-half of ordinary table salt is made up of sodium (natrium or Na^+). The body may lose sodium through sweating, vomiting, or diarrhea. This is one reason why someone who has just lost a lot of sweat may develop a craving for something salty. The body is trying to replace the lost sodium in this way. If sodium is not replaced, blood sodium level can fall (this is called hyponatremia, hypo = too little of natrium = sodium; emia = in the blood).

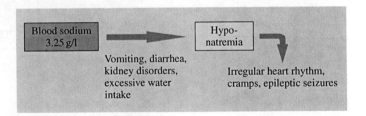

Hyponatremia can cause epileptic seizures, which may need to be treated in the hospital. The treatment of these seizures can be difficult because a rapid increase in the sodium level can damage the brain.

Occasionally, hyponatremia is caused by effects of antiepileptic drugs (carbamazepine, oxcarbazepine) on the kidney. If hyponatremia is mild this does not matter, but if it is more marked the medication may need to be adjusted.

Magnesium

Magnesium (Mg^{2+}) is mainly used on the inside of cells. There are a number of causes of low magnesium (hypomagnesemia). Sometimes the intestines do not take up enough magnesium. In other cases, too much magnesium is passed out by the kidneys.

Symptoms That Occur from Low Magnesium

Mild lack of magnesium	Severe lack of magnesium
irritability, agitation, vomiting, weakness, shaking	tonic-clonic seizures

Magnesium levels can be increased with tablets or a drip. Magnesium is very effective in treatment for epileptic seizures that occur in the case of eclampsia, a complication of pregnancy.

Calcium

Calcium (Ca^{2+}) is required for the normal functioning of the machinery inside the cells and for the lining of the cells (the cell membrane). Small channels in the cell membrane control how much calcium flows in and out of the cells. The blood level of calcium is carefully regulated. If it fails, symptoms of low calcium (hypocalcemia) may develop. Hypocalcemia causes nerve and muscle cells to become more irritable. The muscles may twitch or develop cramps (tetany). This is sometimes confused with epilepsy. More severe hypocalcemia can also cause epileptic seizures.

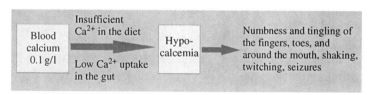

Calcium levels can be increased with tablets or injections. Calcium levels can also be increased by taking vitamin D, which increases calcium uptake in the gut and sets calcium free from the bones.

DISORDERS OF THE DIGESTIVE SYSTEM CAN BE ASSOCIATED WITH EPILEPSY

The gastrointestinal tract breaks down the food we eat into the basic building blocks that the body needs to grow and support its metabolism. The nutrients are taken up by the walls of the intestines and are carried by the blood to those parts of the body where they are needed. Several disorders of the gastrointestinal tract can lead to epileptic seizures. In some of these disorders, treatment is difficult because antiepileptic drugs are not taken up normally by the body.

Celiac disease is also referred to as gluten intolerance, or celiac sprue, or gluten sensitive enteropathy. It is a chronic disorder that consists of an intolerance against gluten. Gluten is a protein in wheat, rye, and barley that can activate the human defense system. The wall of the small intestine can be damaged by the body's attempts to fight off gluten.

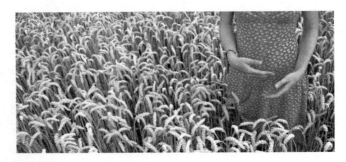

Gluten is contained in many types of grain. It is a type of protein.

The commonest symptoms of gluten sensitivity are related to the gastrointestinal tract: diarrhea, bloating, passing smelly stools that do not flush easily in the toilet. However, gluten sensitivity has also been linked to a number of neurological problems including unsteadiness (ataxia), nerve damage (neuropathy), and epileptic seizures. A blood test can show whether celiac disease is likely.

The treatment consists of a gluten-free diet. This diet may stop seizures if they were caused by celiac disease.

DISORDERS OF HEART AND CIRCULATION CAN CAUSE EPILEPTIC SEIZURES

The brain can only function with a regular supply of blood and oxygen. Any disruption of the blood supply to the brain can cause damage and, ultimately, epileptic seizures.

Stroke

A stroke is caused by an interruption of the blood supply to the brain. One in twenty people who have had a stroke develop epilepsy as a consequence of the stroke. If seizures first occur within 2 weeks of the stroke they are quite likely to stop again (even without treatment).

The epileptic seizures start in the areas of the brain that have been damaged but not completely destroyed by the stroke.

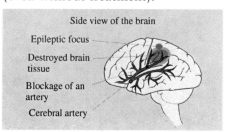

Seizures typically start weeks to months after a stroke, and the stroke does not have to have been particularly severe.

Disorders of heart function

Disorders of heart rhythms may cause blackouts or faints. Usually such blackouts are caused by a sudden drop of blood pressure. Such attacks are not epileptic seizures. Very occasionally, however, a faint can trigger an epileptic seizure.

The nervous system controls heart function. Epilepsy can cause an irregular heart rhythm. In most cases, the problems with the heart rhythm passes quickly and it is not dangerous. However, it is likely that some cases of sudden unexpected death in epilepsy are caused by more serious abnormalities of heart rhythms related to epileptic seizures.

BRAIN TUMORS CAN CAUSE EPILEPSY

Even detailed brain examination with tests such as magnetic resonance imaging (MRI) currently fail to identify the cause of seizures in 8 out of 10 adults who develop epilepsy. However, in a small number of patients with epilepsy, a tumor is identified.

Sometimes it is impossible to say whether an abnormality detected on a brain scan represents a tumor (that is, a lesion which grows) or an area of abnormal brain development (similar to a birthmark on the skin). It is usually possible to get a clearer idea by performing another brain scan after several months, looking for any changes, or by taking some tissue from the abnormal area (biopsy). All kinds of brain tumors can cause epilepsy, but only one in three tumors does.

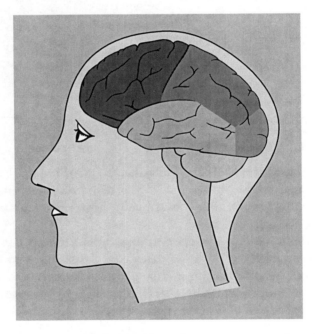

The signs or movements associated with a seizure may suggest where in the brain a tumor may be. Seizures that start with involuntary movements often start in the frontal lobe of the brain, seizures involving hearing things or distorted hearing in the temporal lobe, seizures causing tingling of the body in the parietal lobe, and seizures involving seeing things in the occipital lobe.

The brain is completely enclosed by the skull. There is no room for a tumor, which gradually increases in size. One common first sign of a tumor inside the skull is a headache that persists for more than a week, is worst on waking in the morning, and causes nausea and vomiting. However, one in four brain tumors causes an epileptic seizure as the first sign.

It is important to remember that not every headache associated with nausea and vomiting and not every headache associated with an epileptic seizure is caused by a brain tumor. Sometimes medication used to alleviate headaches can cause nausea and (rarely) epileptic seizures.

Example

Mr. K. has had regular headaches recently. Over the past few days, he has developed dizziness and a feeling of unsteadiness when he walks. Then he suddenly developed jerking in his right shoulder, which he could not stop. An MRI (magnetic resonance imaging) examination showed an area of abnormality in the left half of the brain. His doctor thought that the abnormality was related to a slow-growing brain tumor. He refers Mr. K. to a neurosurgeon. The neurosurgeon thinks that the seizures, headaches, and dizziness will stop when the tumor has been removed.

Tumors with a high risk of seizures are as follows:

Slowly growing primary tumors

Two out of three tumors inside the brain consist of nerve cells or the cells that normally surround and support the nerve cells of the brain (glial cells). Tumors that arise from glial cells are called gliomas (some tumors belonging to this group have more specific names such as astrocytomas—astrocytes are one particular type of glial cell). There are different types of gliomas, some grow quickly (high-grade gliomas) and some grow very slowly (low-grade gliomas). Slow-growing tumors are more likely to cause epilepsy than fast-growing ones. Gliomas do not spread to other parts of the body.

Metastases

Many malignant tumors (or cancers) do not only grow into the tissue around the affected organ. They can also spread through the bloodstream. They may then seed offshoots of the original tumor to other parts of the body such as the liver, lung, bones, or brain. A number of primary tumors can cause such seedling tumors (or metastases) in the brain. There may be single or several (multiple) metastases. Over two-thirds of metastases are caused by primary lung cancer. Other common primary tumors include breast cancer, colon cancer, and melanoma.

BRAIN TUMORS MAY NEED TO BE TREATED WITH SURGERY, RADIOTHERAPY, OR MEDICATION

The most effective treatment for tumors is removal by surgery. Surgery may not always be necessary, for instance, if epileptic seizures are fully controlled by medication and the tumor grows so slowly that its size does not cause any additional problems. Surgery may not be possible if the tumor is close to important brain centers such as areas of the brain important for language or vision. If surgery is possible, it can also stop epileptic seizures.

Brain tumors can also be treated with drugs. These drugs can slow down the growth of brain tumors but do not make them disappear.

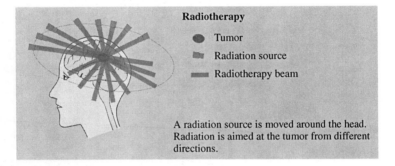

Radiotherapy

● Tumor

▬ Radiation source

▬ Radiotherapy beam

A radiation source is moved around the head. Radiation is aimed at the tumor from different directions.

Another treatment option for brain tumors is radiotherapy.

With radiotherapy treatment, X-rays and other types of radiation are aimed at the tumor to try to destroy the abnormal cells while sparing normal brain cells. Like drugs, radiotherapy cannot make tumors disappear completely. However, it can reduce the size and the number of seizures caused by a tumor. The use of radiotherapy is limited by the fact that radiation can also damage the healthy parts of the brain. One way of reducing the risk of damage to healthy areas of the brain is to aim the radiation at the tumor from different directions. The tumor receives a much higher dose of radiation than the rest of the brain.

Nowadays, a radiotherapy beam can be aimed at abnormal cells that are only a few millimeters away from parts of the brain that cannot be exposed to much radiation. To target radiotherapy with this degree of precision, the exact target area has to be defined on detailed (magnetic resonance) brain scans. The head of the person receiving the radiotherapy has to be placed in a mask that ensures that the radiotherapy beam hits the target area and that the head does not move. Radiotherapy is usually given in daily sessions lasting a few minutes. A course of radiotherapy may consist of 30 sessions over 6 weeks. The commonest side effects of radiotherapy are tiredness and feeling sick.

The treatment options for deposits of tumors in the brain that originate elsewhere in the body (metastases) are similar to options for primary brain tumors. Surgery may be possible for single brain metastases. However, brain metastases are serious complications of cancers of other organs. If there are several metastases, surgery is rarely possible. Depending on the type of the primary tumor, drug treatment or radiotherapy may be possible, but multiple metastases can hardly ever be removed completely from the brain.

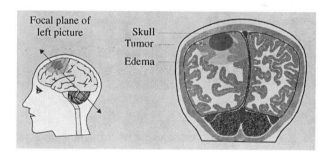

Both tumors and metastases can cause swelling of otherwise healthy areas of the brain. This swelling is called edema and is caused by an increase of the water content of the brain tissue. Often some of the symptoms of a brain tumor (especially headache, sickness, or vomiting) can improve if this swelling is reduced with steroid tablets.

EPILEPSY CAN BE CAUSED BY INFECTION INSIDE THE SKULL

Most infections inside the skull are caused by viruses or bacteria. Bacteria are cells with their own machinery for generating energy, moving or attacking other cells, for instance those of the brain or the lining of the brain (meninges). Viruses are even smaller organisms that essentially consist of an envelope or skin that contains the genetic material needed to produce further copies of the virus. The body's defense system (also called immune system) uses a number of mechanisms (including an increase in body temperature) to destroy both bacteria and viruses. Alternatively, the immune system may be weakened by another infection, poor nutrition, or age, so that a part of the body becomes infected. Antibiotic drugs help the immune system defeat bacterial or viral infections.

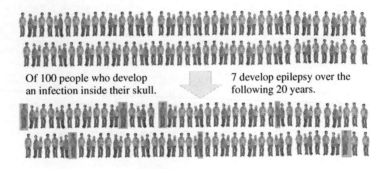

Of 100 people who develop an infection inside their skull.

7 develop epilepsy over the following 20 years.

Infections of the brain itself (encephalitis) or the lining of the brain (meningitis) can cause epileptic seizures. Very often, seizures only occur while the infection is still active. Only 1 in 5 people who have a seizure during the course of an infection develop epilepsy in the long term. All in all 7 of 100 people who have had an infection inside their skull develop epilepsy over the following 20 years. Infections of the brain or its lining are still life-threatening conditions that need to be treated quickly with antibiotic drugs. The signs of meningitis include headache, high temperature, neck stiffness, confusion, vomiting, and a skin rash.

CHILDHOOD DISEASES AND VACCINATIONS CAN CAUSE EPILEPTIC SEIZURES

Several childhood illnesses can affect the brain. The diagram shows some examples. Measles used to be one of the most common childhood infections to cause inflammation of the brain (encephalitis) and epilepsy, although only 1 in 1,000 children with measles will go on to develop epileptic seizures. The risk of contracting measles can be reduced very greatly by vaccination. In fact, in regions in which almost all children are vaccinated against measles, it is no longer a significant problem.

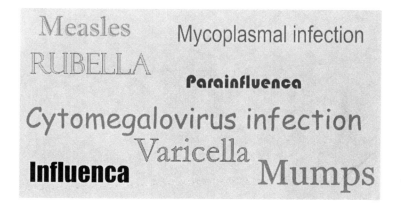

On the other hand, it appears that epilepsy can also be triggered by the vaccination against measles. However, the risk of developing epilepsy is about 1,000 times higher after a measles infection than after a measles vaccination.

It is not clear how vaccinations can cause damage to the brain and epileptic seizures. It may be that they activate the body's immune system, so that this attacks a part of the brain that it should really protect and defend. There is no particular treatment for most childhood illnesses other than protection and vaccination. If seizures develop, they may need to be treated with antiepileptic drugs.

MULTIPLE SCLEROSIS CAN CAUSE EPILEPSY

Multiple sclerosis (MS) is an illness in which the body's defense system attacks the cells (glial cells) in the brain which protect, surround, and insulate nerve cells and nerve fibers. Although glial cells can recover from the damage caused by MS, and the condition does not primarily attack nerve cells, MS can interfere with the normal functioning of the brain. Most people with MS experience signs such as weakness, numbness, unsteadiness, or double or blurred vision. One in twenty people with MS also develops epilepsy. The signs of MS typically come and go at first. However, over the years, most people with MS also develop persistent problems.

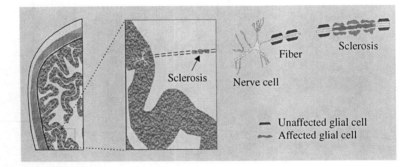

MS affects about 1 in 1,000 people in the United States. It usually starts in young adults in their twenties or thirties, and is one of the most common disabling neurological disorders in young adults.

Epileptic seizures in MS stop spontaneously in almost 1 of 2 cases. They also tend to respond well to antiepileptic drugs if medication is necessary. Epilepsy in MS can be more difficult to treat if the MS is associated with problems with memory, attention, and concentration. People with these additional signs may also be at risk of status epilepticus ("epileptic state," in which one seizure is followed by another).

The occurrence of epileptic seizures does not mean that the MS is particularly severe.

EPILEPTIC SEIZURES CAN BE CAUSED BY MEDICAL TREATMENT

Occasionally, epileptic seizures are triggered in the hospital to be certain about the diagnosis of epilepsy. It may also be necessary to know exactly where seizures start when epilepsy surgery is being considered. However, there may be other situations in which doctors cause epileptic seizures inadvertently, when they do not want to. Seizures can be caused by a range of surgical treatments, medical procedures, or diagnostic tests. Several drugs that are used to treat other conditions can make epilepsy worse or cause epileptic seizures.

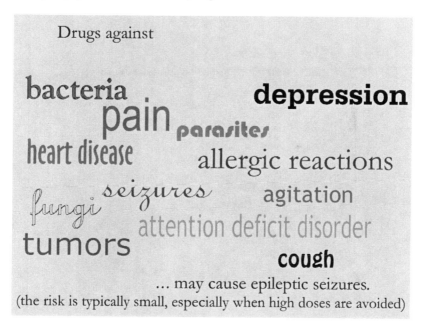

Drugs against

bacteria   depression
pain   parasites
heart disease   allergic reactions
fungi   seizures   agitation
attention deficit disorder
tumors
cough

... may cause epileptic seizures.
(the risk is typically small, especially when high doses are avoided)

When people with epilepsy need medical treatment for another condition, they should always mention their epilepsy and the treatment they are taking for their seizure disorder to the doctor who is advising them about the other health concern. A small number of treatments may not be suitable at all. In most of these situations, alternative treatments can be used that are perfectly safe. Many other treatments may be used with care and if high doses are avoided.

SUDDEN UNEXPECTED DEATH IN EPILEPSY (SUDEP)

"Sudden unexpected death" (SUD) means that someone dies suddenly (within a few minutes) and that the death is unexpected (there is no apparent cause). SUD can happen to anyone; however, the risk is slightly higher in particular groups of people, for instance in people with epilepsy. If a person with epilepsy dies without a clear other cause, doctors may decide that the cause of death was SUDEP ("Sudden unexpected death in epilepsy"). Depending on the presence of different factors, the risk of SUDEP ranges from 1/1,000 to 1/100 per year.

The risk of SUDEP is higher if

- Seizures cannot be stopped by drugs or epilepsy surgery
- The person with epilepsy is male
- There is additional learning disability
- There is excessive alcohol consumption or use of illicit drugs
- The person with epilepsy lives alone
- Antiepileptic drugs are not taken regularly

SUDEP is obviously a serious problem, but there are some things people with epilepsy can do to reduce the risk of SUDEP. If seizures remain uncontrolled, an assessment at an epilepsy center and consideration of epilepsy surgery may help. SUDEP is less likely if antiepileptic drugs are taken regularly and not stopped suddenly. Drinking too much alcohol can be avoided. It may also help if people who have observed a seizure stay with the person who has had the seizure for 15 to 20 minutes to make sure that he or she is okay.

Generally, epileptic seizures are not life-threatening

6

EPILEPSY RESEARCH

KNOWLEDGE ABOUT EPILEPSY HAS GROWN OVER MANY CENTURIES

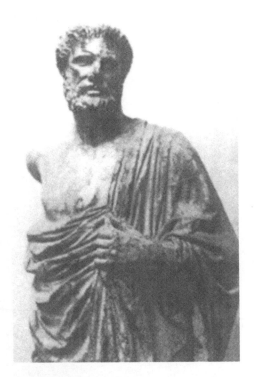

Hippocrates

The word "epilepsy" was first used by Hippocrates over 2,000 years ago. Translated into English, it means something like "surprise attack." Hippocrates described epileptic seizures in a very detailed way, although his insights were forgotten in later centuries. It was often thought that people with epilepsy were possessed by demons or the devil. Treatment was often quite drastic. If treatment killed people, it was said that the demons were too strong. However, some cultures also considered epilepsy a "sacred disease," thinking that people were close to God during a seizure.

Over many centuries, epilepsy was a condition "one should not talk about." People with epilepsy were often excluded from public life. Because epilepsy was not discussed openly, most people knew very little about it. Lack of knowledge and prejudice made life hard for people with seizures. To some extent, these problems still exist today—but we can try to change things. The history of the last 200 years shows how quickly knowledge about epilepsy can grow, but history also shows that such knowledge can be lost again.

BRAIN OPERATIONS WERE PERFORMED IN EGYPT 3,000 YEARS AGO

The picture shows an operation performed about 500 years ago. At this time, some healers thought that they could stop epilepsy by removing a suspected "epilepsy stone" from the head. It is highly unlikely that epilepsy could be improved in this way but some people who had this sort of surgery were lucky enough to survive.

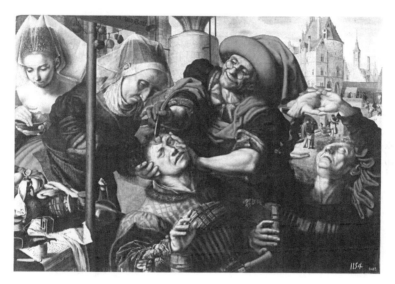

Copyright—Museo del Prado—Madrid—Spain.

Today it is uncommon for someone to get worse rather than better through surgery. The risk of complications has become much smaller over the last 100 years. The main reason for this is the discovery that bacteria cause wound infection. This means that infections can be prevented. Surgery is also much safer now that people can have a general anesthestic for an operation. Modern medicine is the result of many small discoveries that have supported a process of continuous improvement. Of course, not every discovery leads to progress.

EPILEPSY HAS BEEN SPLIT INTO DIFFERENT TYPES FOR OVER 100 YEARS

Some types of epilepsy were first described by doctors who had someone with epilepsy in the family. This gave them the opportunity to observe the illness very closely.

Example

> James Edwin West had his first seizure in 1840 when he was 4 months old. He turned his eyes up and bent his head forwards, initially two to three times, later 50–60 times per day. Whereas only the head had been pulled up at first, soon it was the whole trunk. The head nearly touched the knees. Over the following years, James's physical development was normal but his mental development was slow. His father applied many different treatments. He tried bleeding, cold bandages, laxatives, opium, and even poisons like hemlock. None of the treatments worked. At the age of 3, the seizures decreased and James learned to stand.

James's father was a doctor who recorded his story in great detail. His description and treatment of James's illness was reported in medical journals and books. This means that James's type of epilepsy can now be recognized in other children. Today, it is called West syndrome. It remains a form of epilepsy that is difficult to treat.

In 1932, Hans Berger described the EEG as a new way of studying the brain

Initially, Hans Berger hoped that he had found a method of investigation that would show what people thought. As it turned out, this was not possible. However, it was discovered that the EEG was a very useful tool in the diagnosis and management of epilepsy. The EEG can be used to distinguish between different types of epilepsy, and gives an idea where epilepsy comes from in the brain.

NEW METHODS OF INVESTIGATION INCREASE OUR KNOWLEDGE OF HOW THE BRAIN WORKS

About 100 years ago, the microscopes were good enough to show brain cells. This allowed the Spanish anatomist Ramón y Cajal to develop theories about the workings of the brain. Some of his ideas are still relevant today. Laser microscopes were developed about 30 years ago. They allow us to look at living tissue. The pictures they produce are the result of complicated computer calculations.

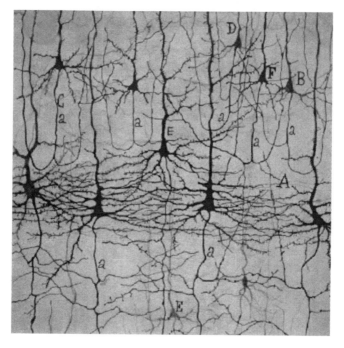

The picture shows a drawing of the different types of nerve cells in the outer layer of the brain, the layers in which these cells are arranged, and some of the cells' processes and connections.

The invention of X-ray machines first made it possible to look inside the skull of living human beings. X-rays are invisible to the human eye. They pass through the body onto a photographic plate. The greater the density of the tissue they pass through, the fewer X-rays reach the plate. Bones are particularly dense. This means that it was not easy to make the brain visible with X-rays because it is surrounded by bone. It was not until 30 years ago that X-ray images of the brain could be produced with computed tomography (CT). A CT picture is the result of the computer analysis of X-rays passed through the skull from different directions.

EACH NERVE CELL CONTAINS THE BLUEPRINT OF THE BODY

The blueprint of the whole body is contained in the core (or nucleus) of each cell. It consists of a set of instructions, which can be read and carried out by the cells. These instructions are held on 46 chromosomes, which may be compared to books on a bookshelf. The books contain 50,000 different instructions (or genes). The instructions contained in the genes have been translated into a language that can be printed out on paper in the Human Genome Project. It is likely that the results of this research will lead to advances in many fields of medicine, including the diagnosis and treatment of epilepsy.

The caterpillar and the butterfly have an identical set of genes. However, some genes are switched on only in the caterpillar; others only in the butterfly. Moreover, the same genes may have different effects depending on whether they are switched on in the caterpillar or the butterfly.

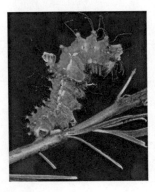 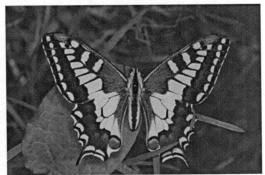

The translation of genes into the language of science can explain only a small (although perhaps important) part of how they work inside the body. One reason for this is that cells only read the instructions contained in a gene from time to time; another is that the same gene can have different effects in different cells of the body. The picture shows how complicated these things are. Using one set of genes, the same animal can live as a caterpillar or a butterfly.

KNOWING THE BLUEPRINT MAKES IT POSSIBLE TO CORRECT MISTAKES

It is likely that genetic tests will make it possible to diagnose epilepsy much more quickly, and to determine the type of epilepsy and the best treatment much more precisely in the future. Genetic tests for some rarer types of epilepsy are already available today. These are disorders in which epilepsy is caused by an error in the set of genetic instructions contained in the cell nucleus. Because all cells of the body carry the whole set of genetic instructions, such errors can be detected by blood tests. However, some people may have such an error in their genes without developing epilepsy.

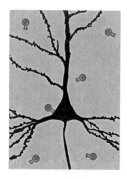

A nerve cell and viruses

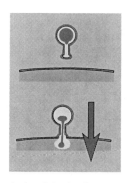

A virus injecting its genes

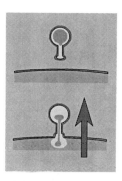

Viral genes replaced by a human gene

One particularly exciting branch of science is trying to develop tools that can be used to fix errors in the set of instructions held in the nucleus. Viruses are one such tool. Their own genes (which could damage the body's cells) can be removed and replaced by corrected human genes. The body's cells can then be infected with the virus, which would insert the correct instructions where they were needed. If the high hopes for this type of treatment become reality, medicine will change completely. There could be special viruses for countless diseases, and many people with epilepsy could be cured. However, it may well take 100 years to get there.

NEW DRUGS HAVE BEEN DEVELOPED

Seventy years ago, few drugs were effective against seizures. These included bromide, phenobarbital, and phenytoin. About 30 years ago, a number of other antiepileptic drugs were developed. These were valproate, benzodiazepines, succinimides, and carbamazepine. Over the last 10 years or so, further drugs have been added to the list of antiepileptic drugs available (oxcarbazepine, lamotrigine, vigabatrin, gabapentin, topiramate, tiagabine, zonisamide, levetiracetam, rufinamide, lacosamide, and pregabalin). The modern drugs had to pass a lot of tests in animals and humans before they could be used by people with epilepsy.

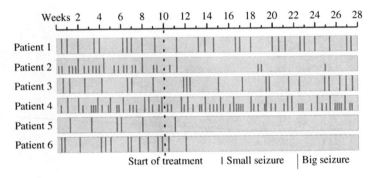

The picture shows seizure diaries covering 28 weeks. The seizures of six different people are recorded. Short lines stand for minor seizures; long lines for major seizures. Patient number 1, for instance, only had major seizures about once per week. From week 10 onwards, patients received the tablets during the drug study. They continued to record their seizures.

Three patients were given tablets containing a new antiepileptic drug, and three patients received tablets that looked exactly the same but did not contain any medication (called the placebo). Neither the patients nor the doctors handing out the tablets knew who was taking medication and who was not. The picture shows that seizures in patients numbers 2, 5, and 6 seemed to improve with the new treatment. After the study had been completed by all patients, it was checked whether these patients had received the new drug.

MORE NEW DRUGS ARE NEEDED

One in four people with epilepsy continues to have seizures despite the antiepileptic drugs available today. We do not fully understand why drugs do not stop seizures in some people. Do they have a type of epilepsy that is particularly difficult to control? Unfortunately, many of the new antiepileptic drugs are not "stronger" than the old ones. They work well in epilepsies that could also be treated with more established drugs, but their effects are disappointing in types of epilepsy that have proven hard to control.

The development of new antiepileptic drugs is based on what is known about the chemistry of the brain. GABA, for instance, is a chemical messenger substance in the brain that is known to reduce activity in nerve cells. Increasing the effects of GABA could stop the development of epileptic activity in the brain. Given that GABA acts on the brain in this way, substances are being developed that could increase GABA activity. Once these substances can be made in the laboratory, their effect on epileptic seizures can be tested.

TESTS ON HUMAN BRAIN CELLS CAN HELP

Operations are the treatment of choice for some problems of the brain, such as tumors. It is rarely possible to remove a tumor completely without cutting out some healthy brain tissue around it.

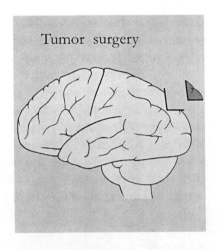

Tumor surgery

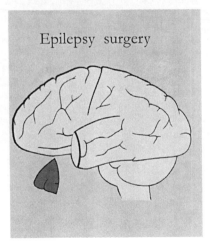

Epilepsy surgery

The removed tissue can be examined under the microscope after surgery. The examination of the tumor tissue determines the tumor type and is important for further treatment. Tests on the tissue around the tumor can help to find out how seizures start. However, such human brain tissue can only be used if the patient has given consent and agrees that some of the brain tissue removed at surgery can be used for research.

In operations for epilepsy, surgeons often have to remove a relatively large area of the brain to be sure that the whole epileptic area has been taken out. After surgery, the removed tissue is examined under the microscope for abnormalities. If they are preserved, brain cells can be kept "alive" for about 10 hours. If patients have agreed that their brain tissue can be used for such tests, the tissue can be used to learn more about how seizures start.

TESTS ON ANIMAL BRAIN CELLS ARE STILL NECESSARY

Albino rats are used for many experiments intended to find out how epileptic seizures start or spread, and how they can be treated. For such tests, animals are anesthetized and later sacrificed.

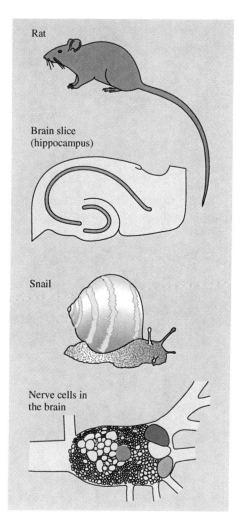

Parts of the brain are removed and cut into thin slices. The brain cells in these slices can be kept "alive" for up to 10 hours. The picture shows such a slice through the hippocampus. As in humans, seizures in rats often start in the hippocampus.

The brains of "lower" animals can also produce epileptic seizures. Some fruit flies (known as "shaker flies") can have seizures when they are exposed to ether. The picture shows a snail and nerve cells from the snail's brain. Some of the cells have been marked. The cells marked in light gray can produce epileptic activity; the cell marked in dark gray cannot. Now the differences between the two cells can be examined. Studying simple nervous systems like that of the snail can help to explain more complicated systems like human brains.

Animals can also have epilepsy.

THE WORKING OF DIFFERENT NERVE CELLS CAN BE STUDIED

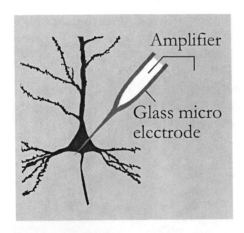

To study electrical potentials in single cells, a thin glass tube is heated in the middle until the glass melts. When the two ends of the tube are pulled apart, the molten glass in the center forms a very fine tube with a sharp tip. This micro-electrode is then filled with a fluid that conducts electricity. The electrode is so fine that it can be stuck into a single cell. It can record electrical activity within this cell.

Using this method, it could be shown that epileptic seizures are caused by abnormal electrical potentials in nerve cells of the brain.

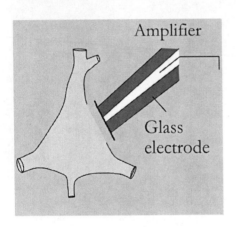

The "patch-clamp" method is another important research tool. It was developed about 20 years ago. A blunt glass tube is pressed against a cell until its wall is stuck to the edge of the tube. When the tube is pulled back, a small part of the cell wall remains attached to it (as shown in the picture). This allows the study of the workings of channels within the severed part of the cell wall.

This method was used when it was discovered that the calcium channels in the cell wall let too much calcium into the cell when epileptic activity starts. In 1992, E. Neher and B. Sakmann received the Nobel Prize for developing the "patch-clamp" technique.

IT IS STILL NOT KNOWN EXACTLY HOW EPILEPTIC ACTIVITY STARTS IN THE BRAIN

We do not know what causes normal brain tissue to turn into tissue that can produce epileptic seizures. It has sometimes been observed that an epileptic focus in one half of the brain produces a so-called "mirror focus" on the opposite side and that a mirror focus can then cause generalized seizures. It is, however, not known how this happens and why it does not happen all the time.

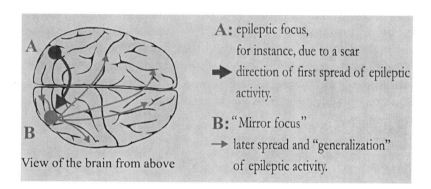

A: epileptic focus, for instance, due to a scar

➡ direction of first spread of epileptic activity.

B: "Mirror focus"

→ later spread and "generalization" of epileptic activity.

View of the brain from above

The two halves of the brain are built in a very similar way. The right thumb, for instance, is moved by a particular area in the left half of the brain. Movements of the left thumb are controlled by the same area in the right half of the brain. Brain centers responsible for the same tasks of the right or left half of the body are closely linked by nerve fibers. Epileptic activity can spread through these connections, for example, from the area in the left hemisphere which moves the right thumb to the area in the right hemisphere that moves the left thumb. This spread could cause a mirror focus. However, it is not known exactly how this mirror focus develops.

There are many gaps in our knowledge about how seizures start and spread. We can differentiate between a person's risk of having seizures, triggers for seizures, and the suppression of seizures, but we do not understand the mechanisms by which these processes happen.

EPILEPSY TREATMENT COULD BE BASED ON THE PREDICTION OF SEIZURES

Most epileptic seizures start suddenly and out of the blue. There is no time for people to ensure that they are safe or to take any treatment that could stop the seizure from developing further. For this reason, taking antiepileptic drugs regularly, and ensuring that there is always a sufficient level of medication in the body, is usually the only practical form of protection against seizures.

For many reasons, it would be better if there was a warning before a seizure that was long enough to give people a chance to make themselves safe and to do something that could stop the seizure from developing. It has been recognized for some time that the EEG can change several minutes before a seizure happens. A number of research groups are trying to improve our ability to understand EEG signals and increase the accuracy with which seizures can be predicted.

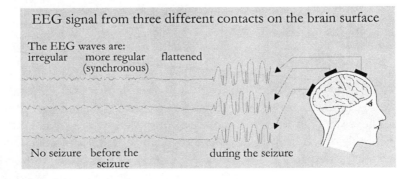

EEG signal from three different contacts on the brain surface

The EEG waves are:
irregular   more regular   flattened
            (synchronous)

No seizure   before the   during the seizure
             seizure

The EEG signal usually produces very irregular waves on an EEG monitor or printer. Some minutes before a seizure starts, the waves flatten. It may be possible to develop a machine that will predict when a seizure is going to happen and that can stop a seizure by sending an electrical impulse into the brain at this point. Such machines are actually being tested now.

WHAT ARE THE LINKS BETWEEN EPILEPSY AND DEPRESSION?

Many people with epilepsy find it harder to deal with symptoms of depression than with their epileptic seizures. Depression can be quite devastating and make people want to take their own life. A number of research studies have shown that there are links between depression and epilepsy, and that depression is different in people with epilepsy. According to one survey of 15,000 American households, depression was more common in people with epilepsy than in people with diabetes or in people without a chronic medical disorder. Thus, depression in people with epilepsy is not just the result of having a chronic health problem.

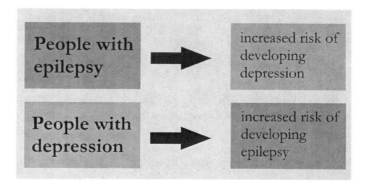

The relationship between depression and epilepsy is probably explained by a shared underlying biologic process. A number of research groups are trying to develop a better understanding of the causes of depression in people with epilepsy. In the commonest form of focal epilepsy, seizures start on the inside of the temporal lobe. This part of the brain contains several centers that are important for the processing of emotions. Learning more about the particular function of these centers may tell us more about the nature and best treatment of depression in people with epilepsy.

MORE MONEY NEEDS TO BE SPENT ON EPILEPSY RESEARCH

There are many examples that show that science and medicine will advance if they are well funded. More money would allow scientists to study a large range of important issues. For instance, there are some disorders of the body's metabolism that can cause epileptic seizures. Although the metabolic problems may be quite different, the seizures they cause look the same. It is likely that different metabolic disorders cause the same seizures in different ways. The diagram shows this more clearly.

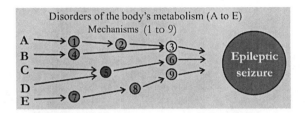

The disorders A–E lead to epileptic seizures through the mechanisms 1–9. We do not know what these mechanisms are. More research into this area could lead to the discovery of new ways of stopping seizures.

An epileptic focus could be treated like some tumors. Many tumors can be treated with particular types of poison. This form of treatment is called chemotherapy. The poison only affects the tumor and not the rest of the body, because it recognizes some special feature that tumor cells do not share with healthy cells. It may be possible to find features of epileptic brain cells that are not present in healthy brain cells. The epileptic cells could then be poisoned and destroyed in the same way as tumor cells are killed by chemotherapy. This could make it possible to cure people of epilepsy with a single course of treatment.

SOURCES

BOOKS

Engel, J., Jr., and T. A. Pedley, J. Aicardi, and M. A. Dichter, eds. *Epilepsy. A Comprehensive Textbook (2nd edition)*. Philadelphia: Lippincott Williams and Wilkins, 2007.

Gumnit, R. J. *The Epilepsy Handbook*. New York: Raven, 1995.

Heintel, H. *Quellen zur Geschichte der Epilepsie*. Bern: Hans Huber, 1975.

Kandel, E. R., J. H. Schwartz, and T. M. Jessel, eds. *Principles of Neural Science (4th edition)*. New York/London: McGraw-Hill, 2000.

Smith, D. F., R. E. Appleton, and J. M. MacKenzie, and D. W. Chadwick, eds. *An Atlas of Epilepsy*. London: The Parthenon Publishing Group Ltd., 1998.

Walker, M. C., and S. D. Shorvon, eds. *The British Medical Association Family Doctors Guide to Epilepsy*. London: Dorling Kindersley, 1999.

Wyllie, E., A. Gupta, and D. K. Lachhwani, eds. *The Treatment of Epilepsy: Principles and Practice (4th edition)*. Philadelphia: Lippincott Williams and Wilkins, 2005.

FURTHER READING

Appleton, R., B. Chappell, and M. Beirne. *Your Child's Epilepsy, A Parents Guide.* London: Class Publishing, 1997, 240. *Answers practical questions about epilepsy in children and how to live with it. Written for people looking after a child with epilepsy.*

Bazil, C. W. *Living Well with Epilepsy and Other Seizure Disorders.* New York: Harper Resource, 2004, 260. *A detailed American paperback discussing many aspects of living with epilepsy and epilepsy treatment.*

Betts, T., and P. Crawford. *Women and Epilepsy.* London: Martin Dunitz, 1998, 84. *Short summary of women's issues associated with epilepsy and treatment. Written for health professionals.*

Blackburn, L. B. *Growing Up with Epilepsy: A Practical Guide for Parents.* New York: Demos, 2003.

Chadwick, D., ed. *The Encyclopedia of Epilepsy.* Merseyside: Roby Education Ltd. 1997, 60. *Illustrated dictionary explaining epilepsy, its investigation and treatment to people with epilepsy.*

Devinsky, O. *Epilepsy: Patient and Family Guide (3rd edition).* New York: Demos Medical Publishing, 2007.

Hanscomb, A., and L. Hughes. *Epilepsy.* 3rd ed. London: Cassell Illustrated, 2002, 80. *A short and illustrated book about epilepsy for people with epilepsy.*

Leppik, I. E. *Epilepsy: A Guide to Balancing Your Life.* American Academy of Neurology, 2007.

Schachter, S. C., ed. *Epilepsy in Our Words: Personal Accounts of Living with Seizures.* Oxford: Oxford University Press, 2008.

Schachter, S. C., ed. *Epilepsy in Our View: Stories from Friends and Family of People with Epilepsy.* Oxford: Oxford University Press, 2008.

Schachter, S. C., ed. *Epilepsy in Our World: Stories of Living with Seizures from Around the Globe.* Oxford: Oxford University Press, 2008.

Schachter, S. C., G. D. Montouris, and J. M. Pellock, eds. *Epilepsy on Our Terms: Stories of Children with Seizures and Their Parents.* Oxford: Oxford University Press, 2008.

Schachter, S. C., and J. Rowan, eds. *Epilepsy in Our Experience: Accounts of Health Care Professionals.* Oxford: Oxford University Press, 2008.

Schachter, S. C., K. B. Krishnamurthy, and D. T. Combs Cantrell, eds. *Epilepsy in Our Lives: Women Living with Seizures.* Oxford: Oxford University Press, 2008.

Wilner, A. N. *Epilepsy: 199 Answers: A Doctor Responds to His Patients' Questions (3rd edition).* New York: Demos Medical Publishing, 2008.

USEFUL ADDRESSES

In the United States
www.epilepsy.com
www.epilepsyfoundation.org
www.ninds.nih.gov/disorders/epilepsy/epilepsy.htm

In Canada
www.epilepsy.ca

In the United Kingdom
www.epilepsy.org.uk/
www.epilepsynse.org.uk

In Australia
www.epilepsyaustralia.net
www.epilepsy.org.au

In New Zealand
www.epilepsy.org.nz

International
www.ibe-epilepsy.org/

GLOSSARY

Absence: Epileptic seizure with brief blackout but no convulsion.

Action potential: Electrical signal used to pass on information from one nerve cell to another.

AED: Commonly used abbreviation for antiepileptic or anticonvulsant drug.

Allergic reaction: Reaction caused by being oversensitive to certain drugs, mostly affecting the skin (red spots).

Ambulatory EEG: Prolonged EEG recording with a portable machine similar to a Walkman.

Amygdala: Part of the limbic system in the temporal lobe.

Angiography: Method of looking at blood vessels using X-rays.

Ataxia: Clumsiness, difficulty with coordination of movement, and staggering walk. Common side effect of anticonvulsants.

Aura: The same as a small seizure (simple partial seizure), warning before a major seizure.

Benign: Likely to take a good course, to respond to treatment, not to get worse, opposite of malignant.

Biofeedback: Method of making the unconscious workings of the brain visible to teach people to influence them.

Brain scan: Painless and harmless method of taking pictures of the brain, either using X-rays (computed tomography, CT) or radio waves (magnetic resonance imaging, MRI).

Callosotomy: Operation in which the connecting wires between the left and right halves of the brain are cut.

Catamenial epilepsy: Epilepsy with seizures occurring before or during menstruation.

Cerebral hemispheres: The two halves of the cerebrum (brain). The left hemisphere controls the right half of the body, the right hemisphere the left half.

Cerebrospinal fluid (CSF): Fluid that surrounds the brain and is not in direct contact with the blood.

Cerebrum: Major part of the brain controlling all conscious brain functions.

Clonic seizure: Seizure with brief muscle twitching.

Cluster: A number of seizures occurring close together.

Complex partial seizure: Partial seizure with impairment of consciousness.

Compliance: Taking tablets as they were prescribed.

Convulsion: Symptom of an epileptic seizure.

Computed tomography (CT): Method of showing the structures of the brain using X-rays and computers.

Corpus callosum: Bundle of wires connecting the right and left halves of the brain.

Cryptogenic epilepsy: Type of focal epilepsy in which the site of the focus and the cause cannot be found.

Cyanosis: Blue coloring of the skin. Sign of low oxygen in the blood. May occur during generalized convulsions.

Déjà vu: French for "seen before." Feeling of unusual familiarity.

Desensitization: Method of reducing the sensitivity to certain physical or mental processes to reduce their effects on the body.

Developmental delay: Slower than expected course of a child's usual cognitive, emotional, or social development.

Differential diagnosis: Range of possible medical explanations for a symptom. Loss of consciousness can be caused by epilepsy, fainting, psychogenic seizures, etc.

EEG: Electroencephalogram. Method of studying the electrical function of nerve cells in the brain.

Encephalitis: Infection or inflammation of the brain. May cause epilepsy.

Epilepsia partialis continua: Condition in which one partial seizure is immediately followed by another.

Epilepsy specialist nurse: Nurse who has undergone special training to advise people with epilepsy.

Febrile convulsions: Seizures in small children triggered by high body temperatures.

Focal seizure: Seizure starting from one small area (focus) of the brain. Identical to "partial seizure."

Focus: Area of the brain that is able to produce epileptic activity.

Frontal lobe: The front part of each hemisphere of the brain.

Generalized seizure: A seizure with epileptic activity in both halves of the brain.

Generic name: Name of the chemical substance used in an anticonvulsant tablet or capsule.

Grand-mal seizure: Major seizure consisting of a period of stiffening (tonic phase) and a period of jerking (clonic phase).

Hemispherectomy: Removal of part of the brain to stop seizures. May be performed in children whose seizures result from brain inflammation, infection, or injury.

Hippocampus: Part of the temporal lobe involved in transferring memories from short- to long-term stores. Frequently a source of seizures.

Hypermotor seizure: Seizure causing wild and uncontrollable movements of the body starting in the frontal lobes, often from sleep.

Hyperventilation: Increased breathing without increased activity, also called "overbreathing."

Ictal: During an epileptic seizure.

Idiopathic generalized epilepsy: Epilepsy of unknown cause and place of seizure onset in the brain with involvement of both halves of the brain from the beginning of a seizure.

Interictal: In between seizures.

Intramuscular: Into a muscle.

Intravenous: Into a vein.

Jacksonian seizure: Seizure in which movements or sensations spread over one side of the body.

Ketogenic diet: Consists mainly of protein and fat and can reduce seizures after some days, especially in children.

Lesion: Area of damage or disease in the body.

Limbic system: Parts of the brain important for feelings.

Lobes: Parts of the cerebral hemispheres.

Magnetic resonance imaging (MRI, also known as MR tomography, MRT): Method of producing pictures of the living brain using magnetic waves.

Metabolism: The making and breakdown of substances in the body.

Myoclonus: Brief muscle jerk.

Occipital lobe: Back part of both hemispheres of the brain.

Oral: By mouth.

Parietal lobe: Part of both hemispheres below the crown of the skull.

Partial seizure: Epileptic seizure involving only a part of the brain (identical to focal seizure).

Photosensitivity: Tendency of the brain to react to flashing lights by producing epileptic activity.

Pillbox: Box for a multiple-day supply of medication with several compartments for each day. Helps people to remember to take their tablets regularly.

Positron emission tomography (PET): Method of producing pictures of the metabolism of the brain.

Postictal: Immediately after a seizure.

Prognosis: Outlook, likely future development.

Provocation: Method of triggering a seizure.

Provoked seizures: Seizures that did not happen spontaneously but had a clear cause, like a head injury or stroke.

Psychogenic seizure (also known as non-epileptic, functional, or pseudoseizure): Seizure that looks like an epileptic seizure but is not caused by electrical discharges in the brain.

Remission: Improvement of illness, when epileptic seizures stop.

Rolandic epilepsy: Benign form of epilepsy starting in the frontal lobe.

Secondary generalization: Seizure spreading from one part to the rest of the brain.

Seizure diary: Diary in which seizures and possible triggers are recorded to observe the course of epilepsy.

Seizure threshold: Likelihood of developing seizures. People with a low threshold are at greater risk of having seizures.

Sleep deprivation: Method of causing lack of sleep to try to provoke seizures in the hospital.

SPECT scan (short for single photon emission computed tomography): Type of a scan that can help to find the source of epileptic seizures.

Spike and wave pattern: EEG pattern typically found in people with epilepsy.

Status epilepticus: Condition in which one seizure is followed by another without recovery in between; medical emergency.

Syndrome: Combination of features of a particular illness found in many people; type of illness.

Temporal lobe: Part of the brain behind the temple.

Todd's paralysis: Weakness of one side of the body immediately after a seizure.

Tonic-clonic seizure: Also known as grand mal. Generalized seizure with stiffening followed by shaking.

Tonic seizure: Seizure with brief stiffening of the body.

Trigger factor: An event that usually starts off a seizure.

Vagus nerve stimulator: Electrical stimulator similar to a pacemaker, which reduces seizures by sending electrical impulses along the vagal nerve.

Videotelemetry: Recording seizures with video and EEG.

INDEX

Multifocal epilepsy, 107
Multiple sclerosis (MS) associated epilepsy, 60, 304
Mumps, 303
Mycoplasma infection, 303
Myoclonic seizures. *See also* Juvenile myoclonic epilepsy
  body movements, 22, 44, 48, 50, 51
  MERRF with, 50
  types of, 23
  valproic acid (VPA) for, 180–181
Myoclonic-astatic epilepsy, 23
Myoclonus epilepsy with ragged red fibers (MERRF), 50

National Institute of Neurological Disorders and Stroke, 10, 11
Nefazadone (serotonin 2 antagonist/reuptake inhibitor antidepressant), 291
Neher, E. (Nobel Prize winner), 318
Nerve cells
  blueprints of body in, 312–313
  in brain cortex, 75
  chaotic firing in brain, 82
  learned self-influence on, 221
  in sensory organs, 76
  skin-brain connection (*See* Skin-brain connection)
  transformation of electrical activity, 77
Neurological examination of brain, 97
Neurologists, 9
Nicotine patches, 251
Nitrazepam, 184
Nobel, Alfred (inventor), 5, 6
Nonconvulsive status epilepticus, 37, 154
Non-epileptic seizures, 100
Normalcy, desire for, 241

Observers of seizures
  as aid to seizure classification, 96
  helplessness of, 18, 95
  seeking help by, 156
  timing of seizures, 95
Occipital lobe epilepsy, 57, 63
Oral contraceptive medication, 213, 265
Organizations for interested people, 11
Overbreathing. *See* Hyperventilation
Over-the-counter medications, 214
Oxcarbazepine (OXC), 189, 294, 314

Parainfluenza, 303
Parents of children with epilepsy
  difficulty of life for, 250
  genetic basis of child's epilepsy, 265, 266

  informing child's teacher, 258, 259, 275
  observation of child's depression, 289
  recognition of child's stress, 137
Parietal lobe epilepsy, 56
Paroxetine (SSRI antidepressant), 290
Partial seizures
  auras, 31, 34–35, 52, 54, 67, 221, 225
  causes of, 29
  complex partial, 30–31, 32, 54, 154, 256
  defined, 16
  phenobarbital for, 183
  simple, 28–29
  simple partial, 28–29, 30, 32, 33, 54
  simple/complex with secondary generalization, 32–33
  temporal lobe onset, 52
  valproate for, 181
Patch-clamp research technique, 318
Pediatricians, 9
Penicillin (antibiotics), 215
Penicillin-induced seizures, 150
People with epilepsy
  disclosure of having epilepsy, 264–265
  driving issues, 282
  equality before the law for, 274
  normal intelligence range of, 242
  normalcy desired by, 241
  rights of, defined by ADA, 278
  wrongness of blanket rules for, 241
Petit mal seizures. *See* Absence (petit mal) seizures
Pharmacists, 9
Pharmacological treatment of epilepsy. *See* Antiepileptic drugs
Phenelzine (MAO antidepressant), 291
Phenobarbital (PB), 164, 182–183, 203, 271
Phenytoin (PHT), 164, 178–179, 185, 186, 265
Photosensitive seizures, 48, 129, 130
Pillbox for medication reminder, 170
Polyfibromatosis (from phenobarbital), 183
Positive emission tomography (PET), 125
Pregabalin (PGB), 193, 314
Pregnancy (of moms with epilepsy)
  drugs in breast milk, 271
  FDA categories, 272
  normalcy of birth, 270
  planning precautions, 265, 269
  risks associated with, 266–268
  status epilepticus and, 267, 268, 270
  ultrasound evaluation, 270
Primary care doctors, 9
Primidone (PRM), 164, 191, 271

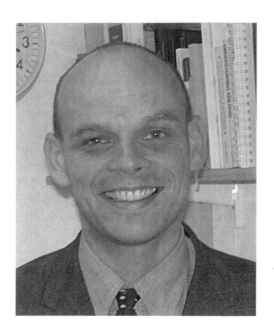

Markus Reuber is Senior Lecturer and Consultant Neurologist in Sheffield, UK. His research has concentrated on how to diagnose and treat seizure disorders and how patients communicate with doctors. He is a council member of Epilepsy Action, the largest epilepsy patient organization in the United Kingdom.

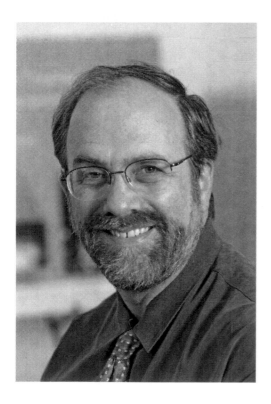

Steven C. Schachter is Professor of Neurology at Harvard Medical School and Director of Research at the Department of Neurology, Beth Israel Deaconess Medical Center in Boston, MA.

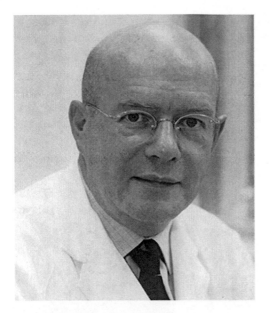

Christian E. Elger is Professor of Epileptology at the University of Bonn, Germany. He heads one of the most important epilepsy surgery and epilepsy research centers in Europe. Much of his research and his work for organizations like the International League Against Epilepsy has helped to reduce the stigma associated with epilepsy.

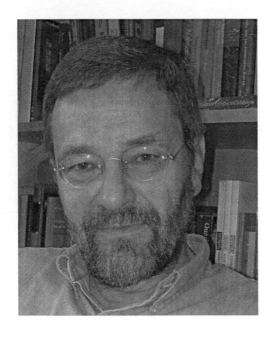

Ulrich Altrup was Professor of Medicine at the University of Münster, Germany. He held the chair of Experimental Epileptology and had a scientific interest in the mechanisms causing epileptic activity in the brain. His premature death meant that he never saw this book in print. He was also unable to complete similar books for people with multiple sclerosis, or people who have had a stroke.